Diagnostic Criteria *for* Neuromuscular Disorders

2nd Edition

Edited by Alan EH Emery

Research Director, ENMC

The ROYAL SOCIETY of MEDICINE PRESS Limited

EUROPEAN NEURO MUSCULAR CENTRE

Royal Society of Medicine Press, London

European Neuromuscular Centre, Baarn, The Netherlands

1997

1 Wimpole Street, London W1M 8AE, UK
16 East 69 Street, New York, NY 10021, USA

British Library Cataloguing in Publication Data
A catalogue record for this book is available from the British Library

ISBN 1 85315 301 X

Design by Nutshell, Newcastle upon Tyne

Phototypeset by Dobbie Typesetting Limited, Tavistock, Devon

Printed in Great Britain by Ebenezer Baylis, The Trinity Press, Worcester

CONTENTS

ACKNOWLEDGEMENTS

These diagnostic criteria for various neuromuscular disorders have, in most cases, been generated by European Neuromuscular Centre (ENMC) Workshops which have been generously supported by the muscular dystrophy associations of France (AFM), Britain (MDG), the Netherlands (VSN), Italy (Telethon & UILDM), Germany (DGM), Switzerland and Denmark as well as the European Union.

We are very grateful to the editor of *Neuromuscular Disorders* (Professor Victor Dubowitz) and to Pergamon Press for permission to reproduce various reports of diagnostic criteria which have been previously published in that journal.

I am personally grateful for the support I have had from Mr Michael Rutgers and the Executive Committee of ENMC (Chairman: Mr Fergus Logan), and Mr Howard Croft and Ms Tricia Dixon of RSM Press. Finally I am especially grateful to Ms Janine de Vries for her exceptional secretarial assistance.

INTRODUCTION

The European Neuromuscular Centre (ENMC) was established some seven years ago with the specific aims of encouraging and facilitating collaborative research into neuromuscular disorders. The majority are genetic and attention has focused on locating, isolating, and characterizing genes for specific disorders, encouraging the sharing and exchange of DNA samples between research groups, and the storing and banking of material. Agreed protocols for assessing the effects of any future proposed treatment are now also being drawn up. But an essential prerequisite of all such work is a precise diagnosis in each case and family being studied. For this reason, priority has been given to establishing diagnostic criteria for these disorders.

This has been achieved through Workshops, nearly 50 of which have been held so far, each attended by experts in a particular field. To date over 600 medical scientists have attended these Workshops mainly from Europe, but also from countries further afield such as the United States, Canada, Australia, Japan, Brazil, Tunisia, Israel and Saudi Arabia. Many of the diagnostic criteria presented in this book have been drawn up by Chairpersons of these Workshops, and have subsequently been published in *Neuromuscular Disorders* where full lists of the participants will be found. With editing, updating and with some additions these various criteria, both clinical and laboratory, are now reproduced here along with a few selected pertinent, but not exhaustive, references.

These criteria are not meant to be definitive but are presented for discussion and it is hoped they will be found useful to both clinicians and scientists engaged in research in this field.

Alan EH Emery
Research Director, ENMC
1997

1 Duchenne and Becker Muscular Dystrophies

E Bakker *Institute for Anthropogenetics, University of Leiden, Leiden, The Netherlands*
FGI Jennekens *Dutch Neuromuscular Research Support Centre, Baarn, The Netherlands*
M de Visser *Dept of Neurology, Academic Medical Centre, Amsterdam, The Netherlands*
AR Wintzen *Dept of Neurology, University Hospital Leiden, Leiden, The Netherlands*

▶ Diagnostic Criteria

Here are presented the diagnostic criteria for Duchenne muscular dystrophy (DMD) and Becker muscular dystrophy (BMD).

Duchenne muscular dystrophy

Elements

1 Symptoms are present before the age of 5 years.
2 Clinical signs comprise progressive symmetrical muscular weakness; proximal limb muscles more than distal muscles; initially only lower limb muscles. Calf hypertrophy is often present.
3 Exclusions: fasciculations, loss of sensory modalities.
4 Loss of unassisted ambulation before the age of 13 years.
5 There is at least a 10-fold increase of serum creatinine kinase (SCK) activity (in relation to age and mobility).
6 Muscle biopsy: abnormal variation in diameter of the muscle fibres (atrophic and hypertrophic fibres), (foci of) necrotic and regenerative fibres, hyalin fibres, increase of endomysial connective and fat tissue.
7 Muscle biopsy: almost no dystrophin demonstrable, except for an occasional muscle fibre (less than 5% of fibres).
8 DNA: Duchenne-type mutation within the dystrophin gene, identical haplotype, involving closely linked markers, as in previous cases in the family.
9 Positive family history, compatible with X-linked recessive inheritance.

Assessment

The diagnosis is definite when:

A The first case in a family:

a age <5 years: (2), 3, 5, 6, 7, (8) all present

b age 5–12 years: 1, 2, 3, 4, 5 (at least once), 6, 7, (8) all present

c age >12 years: (1), 2, 3, 4, 5 (at least once), 8, (or 6 and 7) all present.

B *Another case in the family (according to element 9) complies with the criteria under A:

a age <5 years: 5 and 9 present

b age 5–12 years: 1, 2, 3, 5 (at least once) all present

c age >12 years: (1), 2, 3, 4, 5 (at least once) all present.

The diagnosis is possible when:

a age <5 years: (2), 3, 5, 6, all present

b age 5–12 years: 1, 2, 3, (4), 5 (at least once), 6, all present.

Becker muscular dystrophy

Elements

1 Clinical signs comprise progressive symmetrical muscular weakness and atrophy: proximal limb muscles more than distal muscles: initially only lower limb muscles. Calf hypertrophy is often present. Weakness of quadriceps femoris may be the only manifestation for a long time. Some patients have cramps that are mostly induced by activity. Contractures of the elbow flexors occur late in the course of the disease. Becker-type dystrophy may present with myalgia and cramps, exercise intolerance and myoglobinuria, asymptomatic hyperCKaemia, cardiomyopathy[1] or cognitive dysfunction[2].

2 Exclusions: fasciculations, loss of sensory modalities.

3 No wheelchair dependency before 16th birthday.

4 There is a more than 5-fold increase of SCK activity (in relation to age and mobility).

5 Electromyography: short duration, low amplitude, polyphasic action potentials, fibrillations and positive waves. Normal motor and sensory nerve conduction velocities.

6 Muscle biopsy: abnormal variation in diameter of the muscle fibres (disseminated or small groups of atrophic and hypertrophic fibres), (foci of) regenerative fibres, mostly disseminated necrotic fibres. Dependent on stage and course of the disease, there may be a minor degree of grouping of histochemical fibre types and increase of connective and fat tissue.

7 Muscle biopsy: dystrophin of abnormal molecular weight and/or amount.

8 DNA: Becker-type mutation within the dystrophin gene, identical haplotype, involving closely linked markers, as in previous case in the family

9 Positive family history, compatible with X-linked recessive inheritance.

*When family history is positive (according to element 9) and B is not valid, one should rule as specified under A.

Assessment

The diagnosis is definite when:

A The first case in a family:
(1), 2, 3, 4, 5 and either 8 or 6 and 7 all present.

B *Another case in the family (according to element 9) complies with the criteria under A:
- a the case is a first-degree relative: 4 (at least twice) present
- b in other situations: (1), 2, 3, 4, 5 and either 8 or 6 and 7 all present.

The diagnosis is possible when:
(1), 2, (3), 4, 5 and 6 all present.

DNA Studies

The dystrophin gene was cloned in 1986. Since then it has been found that, in 65% of cases, gross rearrangements (deletions or duplications) have been detected within the gene. Since 1985 carrier detection and prenatal diagnosis have been performed using polymorphic markers within Xp21. The polymerase chain reaction (PCR) technique has revolutionized deletion detection and haplotype analysis. Worth mentioning are the simultaneous amplification of nine exons for deletion detection (multiplex-PCR)[3], the high number of polymorphic CA-repeats for haplotype analysis and the development of methods for point mutation detection. Both the DNA (SSCP)[4] and the mRNA (RT-PCR)[5] methods are now being used. Recently the protein truncation test (PTT)[6] has been developed for visualizing premature termination mutations. Although the latter techniques do not (yet) belong to the standard diagnostic tests, some major laboratories might have facilities to apply them.

Standard diagnostic approach for DNA analysis of DMD and BMD

When a DMD or BMD patient is available for diagnosis, a double PCR multiplex test is performed on the patient's DNA. If a deletion is detected, quantitative Southern blots of the patient's DNA and the DNA of all female relatives are prepared using at least two restriction enzymes – Hind III and Pvu II or Bgl II. This is to confirm the detected deletion, to gain insight into the extent of the deletion and to detect carriers of the deletion. A 'loss of heterozygostity' test for a polymorphic loci within the deletion is a good alternative and may be a better choice for laboratories that do not feel comfortable with quantitative Southern blot analysis.

When no living patient is available for DNA analysis or no deletion is found using the multiplex test, haplotype analysis is performed on the DNA of family members using highly polymorphic CA-repeat markers of RFLPs.

If the DNA of the patient is available but the mutation is not detectable, a cross-over event between flanking RFLPs may occasionally hamper the diagnosis.

*When family history is positive (according to element 9) and B is not valid, one should rule as specified under A.

At present the dystrophin gene is known to harbour some 43 polymorphic sites (GBD-Online Genome Database), ten of which are CA-repeats with a high information content. Routinely used loci include 3'DYSI, STR50, 5'DYSIII, 5'DYSII and 5'DYSI. If necessary, this panel can be extended to other loci, either within or flanking the gene.

In the case of new mutations, the risk of germinal mosaicism[7,8] has to be taken into account.

For a recent review see Ahn and Kunkel[9].

References

1 Muntoni F, Mellis MA, Ganau A, *et al.* Transcription of the dystrophin gene in normal tissues and in skeletal muscle of a family with X-linked dilated cardiomyopathy. *Am J Hum Genet* 1995; **56**: 151–6.

2 North KN, Miller G, Iannaccone ST, *et al.* Cognitive dysfunction as the major presenting feature of Becker's muscular dystrophy. *Neurology* 1996; **46**: 461–4.

3 Beggs AH, Koenig M, Boyce FM, Kunkel LM. Detection of 98% of DMD/BMD gene deletions by polymerase chain reaction. *Hum Genet* 1990; **86**: 45–48.

4 Kneppers ALJ, Deutz-Terlouw PP, van Ommen GJB, Bakker E. Point-mutation detection screening for Duchenne muscular dystrophy by SSCP-analysis of multiplex pcr products by use of the PhadtSystem[tm]. *Am J Hum Genet* 1993; **53**: 1493 (Abstract).

5 Roberts RG, Barby TFM, Manners E, Bobrow M, Bentley DR. Direct detection of dystrophin gene rearrangements by analysis of dystrophin mRNA in peripheral blood lymphocytes. *Am J Hum Genet* 1991; **49**: 298–310.

6 Roest PAM, Roberts RG, Sugino S, van Ommen GJB, den Dunnen JT. Protein truncation test (PTT) for rapid detection of translation-termination mutations. *Hum Mol Genet* 1993; **2**: 1719–21.

7 Bakker E, Veenema H, den Dunnen JT, *et al.* Germinal mosaicism increases the recurrence risk for 'new' Duchenne muscular dystrophy mutations. *J Med Genet* 1989; **26**: 553–9.

8 Passos-Bueno MR, Bakker E, Kneppers ALJ, *et al.* Different mosaicism frequencies for proximal and distal DMD mutations indicate difference in etiology and recurrence risk. *Am J Hum Genet* 1992; **51**: 1150–5.

9 Ahn AH, Kunkel LM. The structural and functional diversity of dystrophin. *Nat Genet* 1993; **3**: 283–91.

This is based on a report originally published in *Neuromuscul Disord* 1991; **1(6)**: 389–91, with permission from Pergamon Press Ltd, Headington Hill Hall, Oxford OX3 OBW, UK.

2 Emery–Dreifuss Muscular Dystrophy

JRW Yates *Dept of Pathology, University of Cambridge and Dept of Medical Genetics, Addenbrooke's Hospital, Cambridge, UK*

At the 1991 ENMC Workshop on Emery–Dreifuss muscular dystrophy stringent diagnostic criteria for X-linked EMD were agreed for use in gene mapping studies. These provide a useful guide for general clinical practice. Similar diagnostic criteria would apply to the rarer autosomal dominant form of EMD.

▶ Diagnostic Criteria

Establishing unequivocal X-linked inheritance in Emery–Dreifuss muscular dystrophy (EMD) requires a minimum of two affected males with obligate transmission of the gene through a female who is asymptomatic or who has cardiac conduction defects or evidence of cardiomyopathy. The diagnosis of EMD in the family can be achieved by having a single case with all the typical features or several cases who between them have the typical features. There is then the separate task of classifying other males as affected or unaffected. Females may occasionally show sufficient clinical manifestations to be confidently classified as carriers, but the status of most at-risk females will be uncertain.

In classifying these criteria, inclusion criteria are indicated with an 'I', exclusion criteria with an 'E' and comments by 'C'.

Requirements for a firm diagnosis of X-linked EMD in a family

Summary

The features which establish the diagnosis of X-linked EMD **in a family** are the presence of all the following (but not necessarily in a single patient):

1 Early contractures of the Achilles tendons, elbows and spine.
2 Slowly progressive muscle wasting and weakness with a predominantly humeral (upper arm) and peroneal (lower leg) distribution, bilateral and approximately symmetrical.
3 Cardiac conduction defect and/or other evidence of cardiomyopathy.
4 Muscle biopsy showing myopathic features or overt muscular dystrophy.
5 Pedigree consistent with unequivocal X-linked inheritance.

Age at onset

C Usually childhood. Onset after the age of 20 years is rare.

Early contractures

I Contractures usually develop before there is any significant weakness. These involve the elbows which result in the arms being carried in a flexed position; the Achilles tendons, so that the patient walks on his toes; and the spine, resulting in limitation of flexion, particularly of the neck.

C There may be extension contractures of the wrist and/or flexion contractures of the fingers.

Muscle wasting and weakness

I Muscle wasting and weakness with a predominantly humeral (upper arm) and peroneal (lower leg) distribution.

I Bilateral and approximately symmetrical. Later weakness of the shoulder, pelvic girdle and thigh muscles may develop.

C Some patients may have facial weakness. There may be wasting/weakness of sternomastoids.

Muscle hypertrophy

C There is usually wasting of the calf muscles.

E Marked calf hypertrophy.

Course

C There is progression of the disease, usually slow.

Cardiac involvement

I Cardiac conduction defect (e.g. bradycardia, extrasystoles, atrioventricular block, right bundle branch block) and/or other evidence of cardiomyopathy (e.g. cardiomegaly, impaired left ventricular function). Such defects may only be evident on 24-hour ECG monitoring. Almost always present by the age of 30.

Evidence of X-linked inheritance

I Pedigree consistent with unequivocal X-linked inheritance, i.e. comprising at least two affected males and obligate transmission of the gene through a female who is asymptomatic or has cardiac conduction defects and/or evidence of cardiomyopathy.

C Two affected males with the same mother are not sufficient evidence of X-linked inheritance and could result from germline mosaicism. If the mother manifests features of EMD the family could be autosomal dominant.

Intellect

E Severe mental retardation excludes the diagnosis.

Serum creatine kinase

C Usually moderately elevated but can be normal.

Electromyography (EMG)

C Myopathic and/or neurogenic and does not contribute to diagnosis.

Muscle biopsy

I Myopathic or dystrophic features of variable degree. Some cases may have focal atrophic fibres resembling 'denervation'.

C Dystrophin is normal.

DNA analysis

C In atypical cases deletions of the BMD/DMD gene should be excluded.

Minimum requirements for designating a male subject as affected in a family with established X-linked EMD

I Any of the inclusion features detailed in 'Requirements for a firm diagnosis' p5–7.

C An elevated serum creatine kinase alone is suggestive but not conclusive evidence of a male being affected.

C Abnormalities on ultrasound or CT imaging of muscles may be useful in confirming that a subject is affected.

C 24-hour ECG monitoring and echocardiography may be useful in confirming that a subject is affected.

Requirements for designating a male subject as unaffected

I Aged 20 years or older.

I Normal serum creatine kinase.

I No clinical evidence of cardiomyopathy.

I Examination by a clinician familiar with the disease shows no evidence of EMD.

Requirements for designating a female subject as a carrier in a family with established X-linked EMD

I Any of the inclusion features detailed in 'Requirements for a firm diagnosis' p5–7.

C An elevated serum creatine kinase alone is suggestive but not conclusive evidence of carrier status.

DNA Studies

Molecular genetic research has focused on the X-linked form of EMD. The chromosomal location of the rarer autosomal dominant form of the disorder has not been determined. Genetic linkage studies mapped X-linked EMD to band Xq28 at the tip of the long arm of the X chromosome[1] and led to the positional cloning of the gene by Bione et al (1994)[2]. The EMD gene codes for a novel 254 amino acid serine-rich protein called emerin[2]. The gene comprises six small exons spanning 2 kb of genomic DNA[3]. To date 26 different mutations have been described in 28 families[2–7]. Most are base substitutions, small deletions or insertions and would result in a truncated or absent protein. Emerin is ubiquitously expressed. In cardiac and skeletal muscle it is localized to the nuclear membrane[6] and has been shown to be absent in patients with EMD. This should provide the means for confirmation of the diagnosis by immunohistochemistry or perhaps Western blotting on blood leucocytes in suspected cases.

References

1 Yates JRW, Warner JP, Smith JA, *et al.* Emery–Dreifuss muscular dystrophy: linkage to markers in distal Xq28. *J Med Genet* 1993; **30**: 108–11.

2 Bione S, Maestrini E, Rivella S, *et al.* Identification of a novel X-linked gene responsible for Emery–Dreifuss muscular dystrophy. *Nat Genet* 1994; **8**: 323–7.

3 Bione S, Small K, Aksmanovic VMA, *et al.* Identification of new mutations in the Emery–Dreifuss muscular dystrophy gene and evidence for genetic heterogeneity of the disease. *Hum Mol Genet* 1995; **4**: 1859–63.

4 Klauck SM, Wilgenbus P, Yates JRW, *et al.* Identification of novel mutations in three families with Emery–Dreifuss muscular dystrophy. *Hum Mol Genet* 1995; **4**: 1853–7.

5 Nigro V, Bruni P, Ciccodicola A, *et al.* SSCP detection of novel mutations in patients with Emery–Dreifuss muscular dystrophy: definition of a small C-terminal region required for emerin function. *Hum Mol Gen* 1995; **4**: 2003–2004.

6 Nagano A, Koga R, Ogawa M, *et al.* Emerin deficiency at the nuclear membrane in patients with Emery–Dreifuss muscular dystrophy. *Nat Genet* 1996; **12**: 254–9.

7 Yates JRW, Aksmanovic VMA, McMahon R, *et al.* Mutation analysis in Emery–Dreifuss muscular dystrophy. *Eur J Hum Genet* 1996; **4** suppl 1: 62.

This is partly based on a report originally published in *Neuromuscul Disord* 1991; **1(6)**: 393–6, with permission from Pergamon Press Ltd, Headington Hill Hall, Oxford OX3 0BW, UK.

3 Facioscapulohumeral Muscular Dystrophy

GW Padberg *Dept of Neurology, University Hospital, Nijmegen, The Netherlands*

PW Lunt *Bristol Royal Hospital for Sick Children, St. Michael's Hill, Bristol, UK*

M Koch *Klinikum der Philipps-Universitat Marburg, Marburg, Germany*

M Fardeau *Institut National de la Santé et de la Recherche Médicale, Paris, France*

▶ Diagnostic Criteria

There are four main criteria which define facioscapulohumeral muscular dystrophy (FSHD) at the clinical level. However, it is likely that the definitive diagnostic test will be at the DNA level; the specificity and sensitivity of a deleted 4q35 DNA fragment at D4F 104 S1 locus is currently being evaluated for this purpose. The four clinical criteria are:

1 Onset of the disease in facial or shoulder girdle muscles; sparing of the extra-ocular, pharyngeal and lingual muscles and the myocardium.
2 Facial weakness in more than 50% of the affected family members.
3 Autosomal dominant inheritance in familial cases.
4 Evidence of myopathic disease in electromyography (EMG) and muscle biopsy in at least one affected member without biopsy features specific to alternative diagnoses.

The more detailed clinical criteria, aimed at a standardized clinical diagnosis, are described below, and offer guidance for genetic studies. Depending upon the results of molecular genetic studies, and in particular the range of phenotype defined by deletion at 4q35 recognized by D4F 104 S1, the criteria may need to be adjusted in the future. Since FSHD is defined here firstly on clinical grounds, the following definitions are understood:

Non-penetrance refers to an obligate gene carrier without symptoms (complaints or subjective findings) or signs (objective phenomena) relating to the disease.

Presymptomatic indicates that a person has no complaints (symptoms) related to the disease but has muscle atrophy and weakness demonstrable by physical examination. (These cases are sometimes called 'paucisymptomatic' in those languages that do not separate the terms 'symptoms' and 'signs' in a well defined manner. Other terms are 'abortive cases' and 'minimally affected patients'.)

Symptomatic refers to patients with complaints and objective findings related to the weakness and muscle atrophy of FSHD.

Clinical criteria[1–8]

Onset

I Onset of the disease is in facial or shoulder girdle muscles. Presenting symptoms usually relate to weakness or wasting of these muscles.

E Onset in pelvic girdle muscles suggests alternative diagnoses; although subsequent pelvic girdle involvement is not uncommon in FSHD.

C Clinically recognizable age at onset is very variable; age at symptomatic presentation is even more so. The mean age at recognizable onset (albeit presymptomatic) is in the second decade. Onset before the age of 5 years, although rare in families, is not uncommon in the more severe proven new mutation cases, and does not exclude the diagnosis. Infantile or early childhood onset requires facial weakness to be present, since a clinical diagnosis cannot otherwise be reliably made.

Facial

I Facial weakness affecting eye closure (orbicularis oculi) and peri-oral muscles (orbicularis oris) occurs in the vast majority of patients. In the absence of facial weakness, a diagnosis of FSHD can be accepted only if the majority of affected family members have facial weakness.

E Extra-ocular, masticatory, pharyngeal and lingual muscle weakness is not part of the disease.

C Facial weakness may be very subtle and is sometimes noticeable by asymmetry of facial expressions only. There is also some evidence that a dominant scapulohumeral presentation without facial weakness may be due to the same mutation mechanism at 4q35.

Shoulders

C The scapular fixators are the muscles most prominently involved. Also the pectoralis major muscles will become affected early in most cases. The deltoid muscles remain unaffected for a long period of time and often have a particular pattern of atrophy, i.e. partial and proximal.

Asymmetry

I Asymmetry of involvement in the shoulder girdle muscle is the rule, usually affecting the right side first.

C Symmetrical weakness and atrophy at presentation is unusual and necessitates increased caution before accepting the diagnosis as FSHD. Asymmetrical involvement of facial muscles occurs frequently.

C NMR, ultrascan or CT-scan may be of help to detect asymmetry of muscle atrophy.

Progression

I Progression is inevitable, albeit at a rate which is highly variable and in some cases virtually imperceptible.

E Regression of symptoms and signs does not occur and would exclude the diagnosis.

C The rate of progression and severity level reached tend to correlate inversely with age at onset.

C Progression of the disease usually includes involvement of abdominal and foot extensor muscles at an early stage; pelvic girdle weakness and upper arm weakness may occur at any time after the onset of shoulder girdle weakness.

C Neck extensor, intrinsic hand and triceps surae muscle weakness is uncommon but can be observed occasionally within families and is not dependent on advanced age or severe involvement.

Severity

C At any age the disease has a wide range of severity. Five aspects of note are:

Overall, between 10–20% of cases have eventual requirement for a wheelchair.

Severity in recognized isolated new mutation cases tends to be greater than in large families.

Presymptomatic cases occur at any age and appear to comprise approximately 30% of all cases in large families.

Once symptomatic, the disease is progressive in the majority of cases. The rate of progression is variable, although faster rates tend to be seen with earlier ages at onset. Rarely, there can be long periods of apparent arrest of progression.

There is broad correlation in 4q35 cases between greater clinical severity and smaller residual DNA fragment size at D4F 104 S1; it is currently uncertain whether this may also be influenced by possible generational anticipation.

C There appears to be no difference in mean age at death between patients and their non-affected sibs.

Contractures

C Contractures and pseudohypertrophy of muscles may be present.

E Severe and diffuse contractures exclude the diagnosis of FSHD.

Cardiac disease

E Cardiomyopathy is not part of the disease. When present it suggests an alternative diagnosis.

Hearing loss

C Hearing loss is part of the disease; it starts with high tone perceptive deafness and may progress to involve all frequencies. The severity of the hearing loss varies between subjects at any age, but tends to be progressive. It is recommended that the results of hearing assessments be documented for several affected members in each family.

Retinal disease

C A retinal vasculopathy with capillary telangiectasis, microaneurysms and capillary closure has been reported in some members of some FSHD families. At present it is unclear whether this is a specific association. It should not be used for diagnostic purposes.

Mental retardation

C A few cases have been reported with mental retardation. It is recommended that investigation of any such case should include chromosome analysis, concentrating on the distal long arm of chromosome 4. However, no causally associated cytogenetic abnormalities have yet been recorded, and haploinsuffiency of the 4q35 region does not seem to cause FSHD.

Laboratory criteria[2,9]

C Serum creatine kinase (SCK) levels can be normal, but are often elevated, though rarely exceed five times the upper limit of normal. Persistently high CK values above this level warrant exclusion of other neuromuscular diagnoses.

C EMG often shows short duration, low amplitude polyphasic potentials. Some neurogenic features such as high amplitude potentials and positive sharp waves are present occasionally, but do not characterize individual families. Motor and sensory nerve conduction velocities are normal.

E Giant potentials are not a feature of the disease.

C Muscle biopsies may exhibit any of the standard myopathic criteria. In addition, small angular fibres are not uncommon and moth-eaten fibres are frequently found. An occasional small group of atrophic fibres may be observed, in which case another biopsy in the same patient or an affected sib is desirable. Cellular infiltrates are not uncommon in FSHD and can be extensive. Their significance is unknown. In these cases, either an autosomal dominant pattern of inheritance or a deleted DNA fragment at 4q35 is required to establish the diagnosis of FSHD.

Clinical inclusion and exclusion criteria within a family for phenotypic–genotypic analysis

Within a FSHD family there may be some members who are difficult to score as 'affected' or 'unaffected', particularly if the significance of a clinical finding can be disputed, or if there are other coincidental neurological abnormalities. Such individuals should be excluded consistently from any linkage analysis. Validation of suggested standard clinical criteria will only be possible once a diagnostic DNA test is confirmed as having full specifity. Phenotypic–genotypic analysis or linkage tests should be based on the following:

I Individuals who have been examined by a physician familiar with this disease and classified as affected according to the above criteria.

I Clinically unaffected family members aged 20 years and over who have been examined as above.

I Unrelated spouses, whether or not examined.

E Any subject whose clinical status remains in dispute.

E Apparently unaffected individuals under the age of 20 years.

E Any apparently unaffected individual with a CK level repeatedly above the normal range in the absence of a proven alternative explanation for this.

Recommended investigations in at least one member of each family included in phenotypic–genotypic studies

The following are recommended investigations:

Fully documented history and clinical examination
Serum creatine kinase
EMG
Muscle biopsy from an affected muscle for routine analysis

Audiometry
Lymphoblast cell line and/or high molecular weight DNA sample suitable for pulsed field gel studies, and tested for persistence of DNA fragment of size ≤ 40 kb at locus D4F 104 S1, following double digestion of DNA with restriction enzymes Eco R1 and Bln 1.

▶ DNA Studies[7,10–17]

In 1990 the gene for FHSD was located on chromosome 4q35. Subsequent analysis by the international FSHD consortium confirmed the linkage, 5 cM distal to the linkage group D4S 171-F11-D4S163-D4S139. In the search for flanking markers a single copy probe was isolated from cosmid 13E. This probe, p13E-11(D4F104S1), recognizes a polymorphic system containing fragments ranging in size from 20 kb to 320 kb. These fragments derive from two non-allelic loci, both containing arrays of a variable number (6–96) of tandem repeats of 3.3 kb monomeric unit size. One locus is on 4q35 and contains fragments of at least 50 kb in unaffected individuals; the location of the second locus is at 10q26, and its fragments can be shorter than 50 kb. Use of a double digest with restriction enzyme Bln 1 in addition to Eco R1 can be employed to capitalize on slight differences in DNA sequence of the 3.3 kb repeat units at 10q26 and 4q35 in order to distinguish between these. The potential of this technique as a specific diagnostic test for 4q35 FSHD is currently being evaluated.

In FSHD patients the 4q35-linked Eco R1 fragment detected by P13E-11 is usually shorter than 40 kb. These 'shortened' fragments differ in size between families but are constant within FSHD families. The significance of these fragments is underscored by the demonstration of the *de novo* appearance of a shortened fragment in over 80% of sporadic cases of FSHD, and by an overall broad correlation between age at first onset and fragment size. The shortened Eco R1 fragments detectable by P13E-11 in FSHD patients, seem to be the result of deletions of an integral number of 3.3 kb repeated units. The gene for FSHD could be contained within the repeated units, or it may be that the repeated units are necessary for adequate expression or integrity of a gene outside this region. Although reports of rare recombinants between the short fragment and the disease in apparently affected subjects may in some cases be best explained by misinterpretation of fragments that are derived from 10q26 rather than 4q35, other recombinant cases, where the short fragment is definitely cosegregating with 4q35 markers, cannot yet be explained satisfactorily. Besides the possibility of coincidental occurrence in the family of a clinical phenocopy of 4q35 FSHD, other potential explanations include the hypothesis that the observed 3.3 kb unit deletion may be exerting either a position effect or a premutation effect on a putative syntenic muscle-expressed FSHD structural gene. Thus, although in most cases the shortened fragment appears directly related to the disease, it is not yet certain if this always remains so.

Worldwide linkage analysis has demonstrated non-linkage to 4q35 in a few families, demonstrating the genetic heterogeneity of FSHD. At this moment therefore, presymptomatic diagnosis can be performed reliably only in large families, or in families where a new mutation can be proved by detection of a new fragment in an apparently isolated case which is not found in either parent. The double digest technique may extend presymptomatic and prenatal diagnosis to smaller families, and perhaps even to single cases, with or without a family history.

References

1 Sorrel-Dejerine Y, Fardeau M. Naissance et métamorphoses de la myopathie atrophique progressive de Landouzy et Dejerine. *Revue Neurologie (Paris)* 1982; **138**: 1041–51.

2 Munsat TL. Facioscapulohumeral muscular dystrophy and the scapulohumeral syndrome. In: Engel AG, Banker BO, eds. *Myology*, McGraw-Hill: New York, 1986; 1251–66.

3 Brooke MM. *A clinician's view of neuromuscular disease*, 2nd Edn. Williams & Wilkins: Baltimore, 1986.

4 Jardine PE, Koch MD, Lunt PW, *et al.* De novo facioscapulohumeral muscular dystrophy defined by DNA probe p13E-11 (D4F104S1). *Arch Dis Child* 1994; **71**: 221–7.

5 Jardine PE, Upadhyaya M, Maynard J, *et al.* A scapular onset muscular dystrophy without facial involvement: possible allelism with facioscapulohumeral muscular dystrophy. *Neuromuscul Disord* 1994; **4**: 477–82.

6 Lunt PW, Harper PS. Genetic counseling in facioscapulohumeral muscular dystrophy. *J Med Genet* 1991; **28**: 655–64.

7 Lunt PW, Jardine PE, Koch MC, *et al.* Correlation between fragment size at DF4104S1 and age at onset or at wheelchair use, with a possible generational effect, accounts for much phenotypic variation in 4q35-facioscapulohumeral muscular dystrophy (FSHD). *Hum Mol Genet* 1995; **4**: 951–8, 1243–4.

8 Tupler R, Berardinelli A, Barbierato L, *et al.* Monosomy of distal 4q does not cause facioscapulohumeral muscular dystrophy. *J Med Genet* 1996; **33**: 366–70.

9 Dubowitz V. *Muscle biopsy*, 2nd Edn, Baillière Tindall: London, 1985.

10 Wijmenga C, Padberg GW, Moerer P, *et al.* Mapping of facioscapulohumeral muscular dystrophy gene to chromosome 4q35-qter by multipoint linkage analysis and in situ hybridization. *Genomics* 1991; **9**: 570–5.

11 Wijmenga C, Hewitt JE, Sandkuijl LA, *et al.* Chromosome 4q DNA rearrangements associated with facioscapulohumeral muscular dystrophy. *Nat Genet* 1992; **2**: 26–30.

12 Deidda G, Cacurri S, Piazzo N, *et al.* Direct detection of 4q35 rearrangements implicated in facioscapulohumeral muscular dystrophy (FSHD). *J Med Genet* 1996; **33**: 361–5.

13 Weiffenbach B, Dubois J, Storvick D, *et al.* Mapping the facioscapulohumeral muscular dystrophy gene is complicated by chromosome 4q35 recombination events. *Nat Genet* 1993; **4**: 165–9.

14 Wijmenga C, Frants RR, Hewitt JE, *et al.* Molecular genetics of facioscapulohumeral muscular dystrophy. *Neuromuscul Disord* 1993; **3**: 487–91.

15 Bakker E, Wijmenga C, Vossen RHAM, *et al.* The FSHD-linked locus D4F104S1 (p13E-11) on 4q35 has a homologue on 10q.ter. *Muscle Nerve* 1995; **Suppl 2**: 39–44.

16 Winokur ST, Bengtsson U, Feddersen J, *et al.* The DNA rearrangement associated with facioscapulohumeral muscular dystrophy involves a heterochromatin associated repetitive element: implications for a role of chromatin structure in the pathogenesis of the disease. *Chromosome Res*; **2**: 225–34.

17 Gilbert JR, Stajich JM, Wall S, *et al.* Evidence for heterogeneity in facioscapulohumeral muscular dystrophy (FSHD). *Am J Hum Genet* 1993; **53**: 401–408.

This is partly based on a report originally published in *Neuromuscul Disord* 1991; **1(4)**: 231–4 with permission from Pergamon Press Ltd, Headington Hill Hall, Oxford OX3 0BW, UK.

4 The Limb–Girdle Muscular Dystrophies

KMD Bushby *Dept of Human Genetics, University of Newcastle upon Tyne, Newcastle upon Tyne, UK*

▶ Diagnostic Criteria

The limb–girdle muscular dystrophies (LGMD) are a group of genetically determined progressive disorders of muscle, in which the pelvic or shoulder girdle musculature is predominantly or primarily involved. The term was suggested to recognize the existence of cases which could not be definitively diagnosed as either X-linked muscular dystrophy or facioscapulohumeral muscular dystrophy in the classifications of Stevenson in 1953[1] and Walton & Nattrass in 1954[2]. Since then, the existence of the group as a separate entity has been questioned because of the overlap of symptomatology with patients who can now be proved to have disorders which are known to be clinically and genetically different. For example, patients with Becker muscular dystrophy and manifesting carriers of dystrophin mutations were frequently diagnosed as having 'limb-girdle muscular dystrophy' before the availability of direct genetic and dystrophin analysis for these conditions[3,4]. Disorders such as spinal muscular atrophy and mitochondrial and metabolic myopathies have also been the subject of diagnostic confusion, as all of these conditions may present with weakness in a limb-girdle distribution.

Even where other diagnoses can be excluded, the LGMD group remains heterogeneous. It is now known that the category of the limb-girdle muscular dystrophies includes a number of separate and genetically distinct conditions, the molecular basis of many of which can now be determined[5,6]. Establishing the precise diagnosis in LGMD may require specialized protein and/or genetic techniques. A number of clinical and general laboratory criteria, however, remain appropriate in order to ensure that the correct group of patients is selected for more specialized study. These clinical and general laboratory criteria therefore form the first part of the diagnostic process.

▶ Clinical criteria

Onset

I In the original description of LGMD, onset of the disease was reported as involving either the pelvic or shoulder girdle muscles or both simultaneously;

the initial symptoms usually relating to weakness in one of these muscle groups. Clinical information available so far from the genetically defined forms of LGMD suggests that onset in these forms is most often in the pelvic girdle.

E Onset of weakness in distal, facial or extra-ocular muscles should suggest alternative diagnoses, though these muscle groups may be involved later in the course of the disease.

C Onset of the disease may be at any age. In recessive families onset beyond the early twenties is rare, but in dominant cases later onset can be seen.

Progression

C Progression of the weakness is inevitable but ranges from very fast to very slow. Preliminary evidence from the forms of LGMD where the genes are known, suggests that there is a correlation between mutation types and severity of disease. Involvement of other systems is rare.

Mode of inheritance

C LGMD may be inherited in an autosomal recessive or dominant fashion. Current estimates suggest that approximately 10% of all patients with LGMD may have a dominant mutation[5]. In the absence of a family history there are at present no clear indications to distinguish the two modes of inheritance (although see comment on serum creatine kinase below).

General laboratory criteria

I SCK is always elevated in recessive cases (at least when the disease is active) and may be used as a presymptomatic test in families where early elevation of SCK has been documented. In some families moderate elevation of SCK has been documented in asymptomatic cases with normal muscle biopsies, and it is possible that in these families carriers show some elevation of SCK. In some dominant families SCK may be normal, and is not normally greater than six times normal[7], while in autosomal recessively inherited cases SCK may be as high as 200 times normal.

I Investigations such as electromyography and muscle biopsy usually provide evidence of non-specific myopathic or dystrophic changes. Muscle CT scanning may also provide evidence of hypodensity in the involved muscles. This may be useful in the differential diagnosis of LGMD and spinal muscular atrophy, as well as determining the exact pattern of muscle involvement.

E The diagnosis of LGMD is excluded by the finding of severely abnormal dystrophin staining on muscle biopsy (providing there are adequate controls for membrane integrity) or the finding of a dystrophin gene abnormality. In female patients presenting as the first case in their family, chromosome analysis should exclude the finding of an X-autosome translocation in association with Duchenne muscular dystrophy. In families with more than one affected boy in a sibship, examination with probes within the dystrophin gene can also be used to exclude X-linkage. The finding of muscle biopsy features diagnostic of a neuropathic process, inflammatory changes, metabolic or mitochondrial abnormalities also exclude the diagnosis.
These exclusions are a vital part of the general diagnosis of LGMD.

Specific laboratory criteria

In patients and families fulfilling the basic diagnostic criteria for LGMD, more specialized tests may now be successful in determining the molecular basis of the disease. Based on the most recent findings about the molecular pathology of the different limb-girdle muscular dystrophies a new classification of the group has been suggested[5]. This classification is shown in Table 1 (overleaf). The genetically defined groups of autosomal recessive LGMD may be subdivided depending on whether or not there is involvement of the sarcoglycan complex[8–11]. In LGMD2A and 2B, the components of the sarcoglycan complex are normal. LGMD2A is caused by mutations in the muscle specific calcium-dependent protease calpain 3, thereby being the first demonstration of deficiency of an enzyme in the products of a muscular dystrophy[12,13]. The underlying molecular defect in LGMD2B is not yet known[14,15]. LGMD2B maps to the same markers on chromosome 2p13 as a gene for a distal muscular dystrophy (Miyoshi myopathy) raising the intriguing possibility that these two muscle diseases, with different patterns of muscle involvement, may arise through the involvement of a single gene[16].

Involvement of the α, β, γ and δ components of the sarcoglycan complex has been demonstrated as directly responsible for four other types of LGMD (LGMD2D, 2E, 2C and 2F respectively[17–21]). Where a mutation is present in one of the sarcoglycan genes it is most usually seen in muscle that the protein encoded by that gene is completely absent or very severely reduced. A secondary reduction in the other components of the sarcoglycan complex is also usually seen. In some of these cases there may be a minor reduction in dsytrophin staining too. Therefore, using protein analysis it is possible to direct mutation analyses in these disorders towards the gene most likely to be involved. In large enough families, linkage analysis may be used to direct mutation analysis towards the most likely gene. A combination of genetic and protein testing is probably optimal in most situations to achieve full diagnosis.

It is likely that not all patients with LGMD will be accounted for by these various genetic loci, and that further mechanisms underlying an LGMD phenotype will yet be identified. However, the current classifications and diagnostic guidelines now available do provide the basis for a rational approach to precise diagnosis in the group.

Conclusions

The current classification of LGMD relies on genetic and protein data. These analyses are therefore essential to achieving a precise diagnosis in any patient fulfilling the base clinical and laboratory criteria.

Current knowledge suggests that all of the various LGMD genes with the exception of LGMD1A are represented world-wide. Further detailed epidemiological studies are however necessary.

A spectrum of disease severity has been observed in association with most of the genetically defined types. Preliminary indications are that the disease severity at least partially relates to the type of mutation found.

Table 1. The genetically defined types of LGMD. Previous nomenclature is shown in brackets.

Nomenclature	Chromosomal location of gene	Gene product	Diagnostic guidelines	Clinical correlates
Dominantly inherited LGMD				
LGMD1A	5q	Not known	Seen in only one large North American family so far	Mild disease: associated with dysarthria
LGMD1B	1	Not known		Associated with cardiomyopathy
Recessive LGMD without involvement of the sarcoglycan complex				
LGMD2A	15q	Calpain 3	Normal sarcoglycan Absence/reduction of calpain 3 in muscle Calpain 3 mutations/linkage to chromosome 15q	Onset usually 8–15 years Progression variable. Correlation with mutation type
LGMD2B	2p	Not known	Normal sarcoglycans Normal calpain 3 Linkage to chromosome 2p	Onset most often 16–25 Progression often slow: some variability Co-localizes with Miyoshi myopathy on chr. 2p
Recessive LGMD with involvement of the sarcoglycan complex – the 'sarcoglycanopathies'				
LGMD2C (SCARMD1)	13q	γ-sarcoglycan	Absent or reduced γ-sarcoglycan in muscle: reduced α, β-sarcoglycan γ-sarcoglycan mutations/linkage to chromosome 13q	Onset 2–10 years Progression from fast to slow
LGMD2D (SCARMD2)	17q	α-sarcoglycan (50 DAG, adhalin)	Absent or reduced α-sarcoglycan in muscle: reduced γ, β-sarcoglycan α-sarcoglycan mutations/linkage to chromosome 17q	Extremely variable severity with onset ranging from early childhood to adulthood Correlates with mutation type
LGMD2E	4q	β-sarcoglycan	Absent or reduced β-sarcoglycan in muscle: reduced α, γ-sarcoglycan β-sarcoglycan mutations/linkage to chromosome 4q	Preliminary evidence of correlation of severity with type of mutation
LGMD2F	5q	δ-sarcoglycan (35 DAG)	Reduction in α, β, γ-sarcoglycan with no mutations or linkage to any of these genes δ-sarcoglycan mutations/linkage to chromosome 5q	Only two families so far reported

Clinical descriptions of the various genetic subtypes are beginning to emerge[22,23]. At the present time, however, distinction between the different types of LGMD is not possible on clinical criteria alone. Collection of reliable clinical data from large groups of genetically defined patients is still urgently needed.

References

1 Stevenson AC. Muscular dystrophy in Northern Ireland. *Ann Eugenics* 1953; **18**: 50–91.

2 Walton JN, Nattrass FJ. On the classification, natural history and treatment of the myopathies. *Brain* 1954; **77**: 169–231.

3 Norman A, Thomas N, Coackley J, *et al.* Distinction of Becker from limb-girdle muscular dystrophy by means of dystrophin cDNA probes. *Lancet* 1989; **i**: 466–8.

4 Hoffman EP, Arahata K, Minetti C, *et al.* Dystrophinopathy in isolated cases of myopathy in females. *Neurology* 1992; **42**: 967–75.

5 Bushby KMD, Beckmann JS. Report of the 30th and 31st ENMC international Workshop: the limb-girdle muscular dystrophies, and proposal for a new nomenclature. *Neuromuscul Disord* 1995; **5**: 337–44.

6 Beckmann JS, Bushby KMD. Advances in the molecular genetics of the limb-girdle type of autosomal recessive progressive muscular dystrophy. *Current Opinions Neurol* 1996; **9**: 389–93.

7 Bushby K. Report of the 12th ENMC sponsored international Workshop the 'limb-girdle' muscular dystrophies. *Neuromuscul Disord* 1992; **2**: 3–5.

8 Campbell KP, Kahl SK. Association of dystrophin and an integral membrane glycoprotein. *Nature* 1989; **338**: 259–62.

9 Tinsley JM, Blake DJ, Zuellig A, *et al.* Increasing complexity of the dystrophin-associated protein complex. *Proc Natl Acad Sci (USA)* 1994; **91**: 8307–131.

10 Campbell KP. Three muscular dystrophies: Loss of Cytoskeleton–Extracellular matrix linkage. *Cell* 1995; **80**: 675–9.

11 Worton RG. Muscular dystrophies: diseases of the dystrophin–glycoprotein complex. *Science* 1995; **270**: 755–6.

12 Beckmann JS, Richard I, Hillaire D, *et al.* A gene for limb-girdle muscular dystrophy maps to chromosome 15 by linkage. *C R Acad Sci Paris* 1991; **312**: 141–8.

13 Richard I, Broux O, Allaman V, *et al.* Mutations in the proteolytic enzyme, calpain 3, cause limb-girdle muscular dystrophy type 2A. *Cell* 1995; **81**: 27–40.

14 Bashir R, Strachan T, Keers S, *et al.* A gene for autosomal recessive limb-girdle muscular dystrophy maps to chromosome 2p. *Hum Mol Genet* 1994; **3**: 455–7.

15 Bashir R, Keers S, Strachan T, *et al.* Genetic and physical mapping at the limb-girdle muscular dystrophy locus (LGMD2B) on chromosome 2p. *Genomics* 1996; **33**: 46–52.

16 Bejaoui K, Hirabayashi K, Hentati F, *et al.* Linkage of Miyoshi myopathy (distal autosomal recessive muscular dystrophy) locus to chromosome 2p12-14. *Neurology* 1995; **45**: 768–72.

17 Roberds S, Leturcq F, Allaman V, *et al.* Missense mutations in the adhalin gene linked to autosomal recessive muscular dystrophy. *Cell* 1994; **78**: 625–33.

18 Bonnemann CG, Modi R, Noguchi S, *et al.* β-sarcoglycan (A3b) mutations cause autosomal recessive muscular dystrophy with loss of the sarcoglycan complex. *Nat Genet* 1995; **11**: 266–73.

19 Lim LE, Duclos F, Broux O, *et al.* β-sarcoglycan: characterisation and role in limb-girdle muscular dystrophy linked to 4q12. *Nat Genet* 1995; **11**: 257–65.
20 Noguchi S, McNally EM, Ben Othmane K, *et al.* Mutations in the dystrophin-associated protein γ-sarcoglycan in chromosome 13 muscular dystrophy. *Science* 1995. **270**: 819–22.
21 Nigno V, de sa Moreira E, Piluso G, *et al.* Autosomal recessive limb-girdle muscular dystrophy, LGMD2F, is caused by a mutation in the δ-sarcoglycan gene. *Nat Genet* 1996; **14**: 195–8.
22 Fardeau M, Hillaire D, Mignard C, *et al.* Juvenile limb-girdle muscular dystrophy. Clinical, histopathological and genetic data on a small community living in the Reunion Island. *Brain* 1996; **119**: 295–308.
23 Mahjneh I, Passos-Bueno MR, Zatz M, *et al.* The phenotype of chromosome 2p-linked limb-girdle muscular dystrophy (LGMD2B). *Neuromuscul Disord* (in press).

This is partly based on reports originally published in *Neuromuscul Disord* 1992; **2(1)**: 35 and 1995; **5(4)**: 337–43, with permission from Pergamon Press Ltd, Headington Hill Hall, Oxford OX3 0BW, UK.

5 Congenital Muscular Dystrophies

V Dubowitz *Dept of Paediatrics and Neonatal Medicine, Royal Postgraduate Medical School, Hammersmith Hospital, London, UK*

The diagnostic criteria for congenital muscular dystrophy (CMD) were agreed at the first Workshop on CMD in May, 1993[1]. The main aims at that meeting were to define the various recognizable syndromes and to establish collaborative studies for gene linkage and further molecular genetic studies. These clinical criteria remain relevant.

▶ Diagnostic Criteria

The term congenital muscular dystrophy has been used widely for a group of infants presenting with muscle weakness at birth or certainly within the first few months of life, in association with a dystrophic pattern on muscle biopsy. There is often an associated hypotonia on clinical presentation but other cases may present with arthrogryposis and associated contractures of various joints. The condition tends to remain relatively static but some cases may show slow progression. Others, however, may have actual functional improvement, pass various motor milestones and achieve the ability to walk. There may be variable respiratory and swallowing problems at the time of presentation and the associated diaphragmatic involvement may lead to respiratory failure in later childhood or adolescence.

In recent years a number of syndromes of congenital muscular dystrophy in association with central nervous system involvement have been reported.

The following clinical phenotypes can currently be defined:

▶ 'Pure' congenital muscular dystrophy

The main features are:

Muscle weakness with hypotonia or arthrogryposis.

Histological changes of a dystrophic nature, often with extensive connective tissue or adipose proliferation, but no substantial evidence of necrosis or regeneration.

Normal or moderately elevated SCK.

Intellect is usually normal.

Brain imaging may show a normal picture or evidence of changes in the white matter on CT or magnetic resonance imaging.

Fukuyama-type congenital muscular dystrophy

In addition to muscle weakness and a dystrophic muscle biopsy, this form of congenital muscular dystrophy is characterized by:

The consistent association of mental retardation which is often severe in degree
A consistently elevated SCK
Consistent structural changes in the brain at autopsy or on imaging
No consistent ocular involvement
Frequent association of seizures with the condition (about 40%)
Survival of most cases beyond infancy and childhood and into adolescence.

Muscle-eye-brain disease

In addition to the muscle weakness and associated dystrophic changes in the muscle, there is consistent ocular and central nervous system involvement. There is associated mental retardation which is often severe.

The most consistent ocular abnormality is severe myopia but there may also be strabismus, glaucoma, lens opacity, retinal atrophy and optic atrophy. Epilepsy is also commonly associated and the EEG is always abnormal after the age of one year. Hydrocephalus is present in the majority of cases. The SCK may be normal within the first year, but is always elevated thereafter.

Walker-Warburg syndrome

This syndrome is characterized by structural changes and associated mental retardation in addition to the muscle weakness and dystrophic changes.

The consistent central nervous system abnormalities on imgaging are a type II lissencephaly, comprising variable gyral malformations, together with an abnormally thick cortex and decreased interdigitations between the white matter and cortex. There may also be other structural changes within the nervous system. Ocular malformations are also common but are thought to be less severe and less consistent than in muscle-eye-brain disease.

There is divergence of opinion as to whether the Walker-Warburg syndrome and muscle-eye-brain disease constitute one entity with variable severity, or whether they represent two separate entities in view of the more striking ocular involvement in muscle-eye-brain disease. There is certainly some degree of overlap in the structural changes within the central nervous system.

DNA and Protein Studies

By the time of the second Workshop in April, 1994[2], the gene for Fukuyama CMD had been located on chromosome 9q, and a deficiency of a protein, the laminin alpha-2 chain of merosin, had been discovered in about 40% of the cases of classical CMD. Further studies showed that this was indeed a primary deficiency, and that these cases linked to the locus of the corresponding gene (LAMA2) on chromosome 6q. It also became clear once the classical cases were subdivided into merosin deficient and merosin positive, that the merosin deficient group comprised a much more severe phenotype, usually with inability to walk unaided, in contrast to the merosin-positive group, most of whom achieved independent walking. In addition the cases that had shown increased signal in the white matter in T2-weighted magnetic resonance imaging of the brain were also consistently merosin deficient.

At the recent third Workshop in March, 1996[3], mutations in the LAMA2 gene were reported in a small number of merosin-deficient cases to date. With the more routine screening for merosin in all dystrophic biopsies, without deficiency of dystrophin or the sarcoglycans, a number of atypical cases of CMD with later onset or milder phenotype have also been recognized.

An important new development, also reported at the third Workshop, was the discovery of a deficit in the protein alpha-actinin 3, in a small number of cases of merosin-positive CMD. It is not yet known whether this is a primary or a secondary deficit, and what proportion of cases of merosin-positive CMD it is associated with.

With regard to the Walker–Warburg syndrome and muscle–eye–brain disease, it has not yet been possible to establish a gene location, and whether they constitute two separate entities or not, mainly due to the relative rarity of these two syndromes and availability of informative families. The data suggest that they are not linked to either chromosome 6q or 9q, so that they are probably distinct from classical CMD and Fukuyama CMD (Table 1).

Table 1. The congenital muscular dystrophies.

Clinical type	Main clinical features	Protein deficiency	Gene location	Gene mutations
Classical CMD	No intellectual impairment No structural abnormality in brain	Merosin-deficiency (primary)	6q	+
		Merosin-positive α-actinin 3 deficiency	?	
		Merosin-positive	?	
Fukuyama CMD	Associated mental retardation and structural brain abnormality	Partial merosin deficiency (secondary)	9q	
Muscle–eye–brain disease	Mental retardation Structural brain changes Ocular abnormalities			
Walker–Warburg syndrome	Mental retardation Lissencephaly II Eye changes			

References

1 Dubowitz V. Workshop report: 22nd ENMC sponsored Workshop on congenital muscular dystrophy. *Neuromuscul Disord* 1994; **4**: 75–81.

2 Dubowitz V, Fardeau M. Workshop report: 27th ENMC sponsored international Workshop: congenital muscular dystrophy. *Neuromuscul Disord* 1995; **5(3)**: 253–8.

3 Dubowitz V. Workshop report: 41st ENMC sponsored international Workshop: congenital muscular dystrophy. *Neuromuscul Disord* 1996; **6(4)**: 295–301.

This is based on reports originally published in *Neuromuscul Disord* 1994; **4(1)**: 75–81, 1995; **5(3)**: 253–8 and 1996; **6(4)**: 295–301 with permission from Pergamon Press Ltd, Headington Hill Hall, Oxford

6 Myotonic Dystrophy (Steinert's Disease)

HG Brunner *Dept of Anthropogenetics, University Hospital Nijmegen, Nijmegen, The Netherlands*

FGI Jennekens *Dutch Neuromuscular Research Support Centre, Baarn, The Netherlands*

HJM Smeets *Dept of Anthropogenetics, University Hospital Nijmegen, Nijmegen, The Netherlands*

M de Visser *Dept of Neurology, Academic Medical Centre, Amsterdam, The Netherlands*

AR Wintzen *Dept of Neurology, University Hospital, Leiden, The Netherlands*

▶ Diagnostic Criteria

With regard to the diagnostic criteria for myotonic dystrophy, the clinical picture depends on the age at onset.

a Congenital (1) and early childhood myotonic dystrophy (2), age <10 years.
b Juvenile/adult (classical) myotonic dystrophy, age 10–50 years.
c Minimal myotonic dystrophy, age >50 years.

Elements

a1 Congenital myotonic dystrophy

1 Stillbirth or generalized severe muscular weakness (including the face) and hypotonia with sucking, swallowing and sometimes respiratory insufficiency. Absence of tendon reflexes. Club feet.
2 Symptoms of myotonic dystrophy (see b) in the mother.
3 Amplification (>45) of a trinucleotide repeat unit in the myotonic dystrophy gene on chromosome 19.

a2 Early childhood myotonic dystrophy

1 Mental retardation.
2 Generalized weakness, especially of the face and distal limbs; myotonia starts usually between the ages of 5 and 10 years.
3 Electroymyography*: myotonic volleys in several muscles.
4 Symptoms of myotonic dystrophy in one of the parents.

*Electromyography: myotonic volleys ('dive bomber') resemble repetitive denervation potentials with inconstant frequency 20–120 Hz, duration at least 0.5 s. Examination of mm. orbicularis oris, masseter, thenar, tibialis anterior.

5 Amplification (>45) of a trinucleotide repeat unit in the myotonic dystrophy gene on chromosome 19.

b Juvenile/adult (classical) mytonic dystrophy

1 Myotonia of grip and/or percussion myotonia of thenar muscle.
2 Weakness of one or more of the following: m. orbicularis oculi., pharyngeal muscles, distal limb muscles. Atrophy of masticatory muscles and/or distal limb muscles may be obvious.
3 Cortical cataract‡ (slit lamp examination mandatory).
4 Electromyography*: myotonic volleys in several muscles.
5 Positive family history compatible with autosomal dominant inheritance.
6 Amplification (>45) of a trinucleotide repeat unit in the myotonic dystrophy gene on chromosome 19.

c Minimal myotonic dystrophy

1 Cortical cataract‡ Rarely neuromuscular symptoms (see b).
2 Electromyography*: myotonic volleys in several muscles.
3 Positive family history compatible with autosomal dominent inheritance.
4 Amplification (>45) of a trinucleotide repeat unit in the myotonic dystrophy gene on chromosome 19.

Asymptomatic heterozygotes occur, even in old age.

Assessment

The diagnosis is definite as shown in Table 1.

Table 1. *Assessment of myotonic dystrophy. (§ When family history is positive and B is not valid, one should rule as under A.)*

A	First case in the family	B§	There is a first-degree relative who complies with the criteria under A
a1	1, 2, (3) all present		1, 2 (3) all present
a2	(1), 2, (3), 4, (5) all present		(1), 2, (3), 4, (5) all present
b	One of 1–4, (5) and 6		1, 2 2 3 4 or 6 present
c	>1 element and 4 present		1 or 2 or 4 present

‡Cataract should be cortical, assessed by experienced ophthalmologist with slit lamp and should not be used as criterion if no first-degree family member is affected.
*Electromyography: myotonic volleys ('dive bomber') resemble repetitive denervation potentials with inconstant frequency 20–120 Hx, duration at least 0.5 s. Examination of mm. orbicularis oris, masseter, thenar, tibialis anterior.

▶ DNA Studies

Myotonic dystrophy or dystrophia myotonica (DM) is caused by an increased number of CTG trinucleotide repeats located in the 3′-untranslated region of the putative DM gene. This gene has been termed DM-kinase (or myotonin-kinase) because of similarities to a class of genes that encode serine/threonine kinases.

Molecular diagnosis of DM is possible by DNA analysis of various tissues, usually blood cells, muscle chorionic villus or amnion cells. The DM mutation is detected either by Southern blotting and hybridization with a DNA probe or by polymerase chain reaction (PCR) of the relevant DNA fragment.

The number of CTG trinucleotides on normal chromosomes ranges from 3 to 30. When the CTG repeat number exceeds 40, the DNA repeat seqence is unstable[1] and the number of repeats tends to increase on parent-to-child transmission. A decrease in CTG number occurs more rarely. Unstable repeats of 40 to approximately 100 CTG trinucleotides are often associated with cataract but muscular symptoms are very rare. Such repeats nearly always increase on transmission to the next generation (so-called "anticipation") and this increase is most marked when tramission is through a female. Larger repeats found in offspring may range from less than 100 to several thousand CTG trinucleotides. The number of CTG trinucleotides correlates broadly with age at onset and severity of symptoms. However, genotype/phenotype correlates are currently too imprecise to allow precise DNA-based prognosis.

For recent reviews see Harley *et al*[1] and Harper and Rüdel[2].

References

1 Harley HG, Rundle SA, MacMillan JC, *et al.* Size of the unstable CTG repeat sequence in relation to phenotype and parental transmission in myotonic dystrophy. *Am J Hum Genet* 1993; 52: 1164–74.

2 Harper PS, Rüdel R. Myotonic dystrophy. In: Engel AG and Franzini-Armstrong C (editors) *Myology, basic and clinical.* New York: McGraw-Hill Inc, 1994: 1192–219.

This is based on a report originally published in *Neuromuscul Disord* 1991; 1(6):389–91 with permission from Pergamon Press Ltd, Headington Hill Hall, Oxford OX3 0BW, UK

7 Non-dystrophic Myotonias and Periodic Paralyses

F Lehmann-Horn and R Rüdel *Dept of Physiology, University of Ulm, Ulm, Germany*

▶ Diagnostic Criteria

Since the genes and the gene products are known in the principal diseases of non-dystrophic mytonias and periodic paralyses, and since an increasing number of molecular biological laboratories have the relevant genetic markers available, an exact diagnosis can be made by the identification of the mutation. At present, many laboratories are engaged in correlating the clinical symptoms of their individual families with the various mutations and, therefore, a precise statement of the clinical diagnostic criteria remains useful[1,2].

It is important to state that myotonia, i.e. muscle stiffness, is a **symptom** that can be present in both muscle Cl^- and Na^+ channel diseases (and, of course, also in myotonic dystrophy, proximal myotonic myopathy and Schwartz-Jampel syndrome). The myotonia is best assessed as **myotonic runs** in the electromyogram. Diagnostic differentiation of the various diseases on the mere basis of these runs is not dependable. Muscle biopsy is usually not helpful for establishing the diagnosis.

The class of Cl^- channel diseases comprises dominant myotonia congenita (Thomsen) and recessive generalized myotonia (Becker). The term **myotonia congenita** should only be reserved for these Cl^- channel diseases.

The class of Na^+ channel diseases encompasses hyperkalaemic periodic paralysis (HyperPP), normokalaemic periodic paralysis (NormoPP), paramyotonia congenita (PC) and potassium-aggravated myotonia (PAM). Although the key symptoms, namely attacks of muscle weakness and episodes of muscle stiffness, are known to overlap to various degrees, it makes sense from a clinical point of view to maintain the differentiation between HyperPP (identical with Gamstorp's adynamia episodica hereditaria) and PC, because preventive measures are different for the two syndromes. HyperPP also implies a possible prognosis of progressive permanent weakness that is not a feature of PC. In potassium-aggravated myotonia the key symptom is muscle stiffness that resembles the myotonia in myotonia congenita. This myotonia may be mild (myotonia fluctuans), moderate or severe (myotonia permanens). Hypokalaemic periodic paralysis, the only disease in this group not associated with myotonia, is a Ca^{++} channel disease.

Dominant myotonia congenita

The usual (but rare) form is Thomsen's disease[2,3,4]. There is also a form that is distinguished by very mild myotonia (De Jong's myotonia levior). It is caused by an allelic mutation in the muscle chloride channel gene[5].

Family history

Autosomal dominant inheritance; 100% penetrance.

Age at onset

From birth to early childhood.

Clinical signs

Muscle stiffness, particularly after rest, muscle function improving with continuing exercise (warm up). Myotonia fluctuates only slightly during lifetime; there is no progression and muscle hypertrophy is frequent. Although patients with myotonia congenita, when asked, often state that their stiffness increases in the cold, this cannot be substantiated with objective measurements of muscle relaxation times.

Clinical signs which must not be mistaken. There are cases of Na^+ channel disease having myotonia without any weakness (PAM). The myotonia may exist without cooling. Before the advent of molecular biology, these cases were misdiagnosed as forms of myotonia congenita.

Recessive generalized myotonia

Many loss-of-function mutations in the muscle chloride channel gene can cause the same clinical picture[4,6,7,8].

Family history

Autosomal recessive inheritance. Some of the heterozygous carriers show myotonic runs in the EMG. Such cases must not be confused with dominant myotonia, and sometimes molecular biology is required to differentiate this from myotonic dystrophy.

Age at onset

Occasionally present in early childhood, usually the first decade of life, in some cases not before the end of the second decade, and even progression of symptoms into the third decade of life.

Clinical signs

Muscle stiffness, particularly after rest, muscle function improving with continuing exercise (warm up). In many patients marked transient weakness after rest which improves during several minutes of continued exercise. Weakness is more pronounced in the upper extremities, stiffness is more pronounced in the legs. In many cases hip and leg muscles are hypertrophied. The signs are usually progressive for a few years after their first appearance and then remain stable for the rest of life.

Clinical signs which must not be mistaken. The well-known phenomenon of anticipation in myotonic dystrophy may lead to a familial constellation suggesting recessive inheritance and, as a consequence, may lead to the spurious diagnosis of recessive generalized myotonia. On the other hand, misinterpretation of the transient weakness may lead to the spurious diagnosis of myotonic dystrophy. In older patients with recessive generalized myotonia muscle biopsies may show a morphologic pattern that can be misdiagnosed as myotonic dystrophy.

Paramyotonia congenita

The classical form was described by Eulenburg and independently by Rich. Several mutations in the Na^+ channel gene result in the classical clinical picture[9,10].

Family history

Autosomal dominant inheritance; 100% penetrance.

Age at onset

From birth.

Clinical signs

Muscle stiffness increasing with exercise (paradoxical myotonia). In many families paramyotonia is dramatically increased when the muscles are exercised in the cold. Recovery from weakness may last several hours.
Some families present consistently cold- and exercise-induced stiffness without weakness. These are often misdiagnosed as having myotonia congenita.

Variability of signs. There are families where affected members present with the classical symptoms of paramyotonia congenita and also often experience attacks of hyperkalaemic paralysis. The presentation of both sets of symptoms in severe form was termed paralysis periodica paramyotonica (PPP) by PE Becker; however, a continuum seems to exist, with PPP families and families having 'pure' paramyotonia congenita presenting the two extremes. The severity of stiffness is not the same in all paramyotonia families.

Clinical signs which must not be mistaken. Permanent weakness is not observed in paramyotonia congenita.

Hyperkalaemic periodic paralysis

Several mutations in the Na^+ channel gene may lead to the classical clinical picture.

Family history

Autosomal dominant inheritance; complete penetrance, but severity is very variable.

Age at onset

Early childhood to second decade of life.

Clinical signs

Attacks of weakness, usually in the morning, lasting from 10 min to 1 h or so, very rarely up to 1–2 days. Some patients experience only a few attacks of weakness in their lifetime, others have attacks of generalized weakness almost every day. During the attacks, serum K^+ is elevated to upper normal levels or above. Myotonic stiffness is not observed. Rest after exercise, fasting, or oral intake of K^+ are very efficient in precipitating attacks (provocative tests). Some patients always show slight signs of mytonia between and at the beginning of attacks; others show signs of paramyotonia; in a third category myotonic signs are absent.

Clinical signs which must be not mistaken. At the end of a paralytic attack, serum K^+ can fall below the normal level. A blood sample taken during this time can suggest hypokalaemic periodic paralysis.

Normokalaemic periodic paralysis

Very few families have been described. Attacks can last several days without an increase of the serum K^+ concentration. Since it was shown for one family that the Na^+ channel gene is mutated at a locus (Thr704) that causes HyperPP in other families we suggest that the form of periodic paralysis without hyperkalaemia is a variant of HyperPP.

Potassium-aggravated myotonia (PAM)

So far five different mutations in the Na^+ channel gene have been described[11,12,13].

Family history

Autosomal dominant inheritance.

Clinical signs

Myotonia fluctuans

Muscle stiffness, which may fluctuate from day to day, is provoked by exercise ('delayed-onset myotonia'). Ingestion of potassium aggravates myotonia but does not induce weakness as in hyperkalaemic periodic paralysis. Also other depolarizing agents such as suxamethonium can induce or aggravate myotonia so that severe ventilation problems may occur during general anaesthesia if patient and anaesthesiologist are unaware of the condition. Even in the absence of clinical myotonia, latent myotonia can be consistently recorded by the use of electromyography. In acetazolamide-responsive myotonia, also described as atypical myotonia congenita, the muscle stiffness also fluctuates and, in addition, muscle pain is induced by exercise.

Myotonia permanens

Persistent generalized myotonia and muscle hypertrophy, particularly in the neck and shoulder. Attacks of severe muscle stiffness of the thoracic muscles may be life-threatening due to impaired ventilation, in particular in children. Since the myotonia is so severe and further aggravated by depolarizing agents, potassium must never be administered as a diagnostic tool.

Hypokalaemic periodic paralysis

Two mutations in the gene (CACLN1A3) encoding the L-type calcium channel (DHP receptor) $\alpha 1$ subunit cause the clinical picture in more than 50% of the families[14,15,16].

Family history

Autosomal dominant trait with reduced penetrance in women (the male to female ratio is 3–4 to 1).

Age of onset

Severe cases present in early childhood, about 60% present before age 16, and mild cases as late as the third decade of life.

Clinical signs

Attacks of weakness, usually in the second half of the night or in the early morning. Initially the attacks are infrequent but after a few months or years they increase in frequency, and eventually may recur daily. An attack may range in severity from slight temporary weakness of an isolated muscle group to generalized paralysis. Usually strength gradually increases as the day passes. Occasionally the weakness lasts 2 to 3 days. The trigger for a nocturnal attack is often strenuous physical activity or a carbohydrate-rich meal on the preceding day. During the day, attacks can be provoked or worsened by high carbohydrate and high sodium intake, and by excitement. Slight physical activity can sometimes prevent or delay mild attacks. During major attacks, the serum potassium decreases and may cause sinus bradycardia and ECG signs of hypokalaemia. Neither clinical nor electrical myotonia is present. Independently of the severity and frequency of the paralytic attacks, 30% of the patients develop a progressive proximal myopathy with permanent residual weakness.

DNA Studies

Electrophysiology has shown that the muscle stiffness in dominant myotonia congenita (Thomsen) and in recessive generalized myotonia (Becker) is caused by a reduction of the Cl^- conductance of the muscle fibre membrane. After the CHLCN1 gene encoding the muscular Cl^- channel was localized on chromosome 7q32-ter, linkage was quickly established for both Thomsen and Becker families.

Several dominant or recessive allelic mutations have been discovered. Electrophysiology has suggested and molecular biology has proved that paramyotonia congenita, hyper- and normokalaemic periodic paralysis, as well as PAM are caused by point mutations in the gene encoding the α subunit of the Na^+ channel in adult human skeletal muscle, located on chromosome 17q23. Nineteen different mutations have been described. After a systematic genome-wide search had demonstrated linkage of hypokalaemic periodic paralysis to chromosome 1q31-32 and co-segregation with the gene encoding the L-type calcium channel (DHP receptor) $\alpha 1$ subunit, sequencing of cDNA derived from muscle biopsies of patients has revealed three mutations so far. As shown by screening of genomic DNA, the majority of the families carry either the Arg-528-His or the Arg-1239-His substitution.

▶ References

1 Hoffman EP, Lehmann-Horn F, Rüdel R. Overexcited or inactive: Ion channels in muscle disease. *Cell* 1995; **80**: 681–6.

2 Lehmann-Horn F, Rüdel R. Molecular pathophysiology of voltage-gated ion channels. *Rev Physiol Biochem Pharmacol* 1996; **128**: 197–268.

3 George AL Jr, Sloan-Brown K, Fenichel GM, *et al.* Nonsense and missense mutations of the muscle chloride channel gene in patients with myotonia congenita. *Hum Mol Genet* 1994; **3**: 2071–2.

4 Meyer-Kleine C, Steinmeyer K, Ricker K, *et al.* Spectrum of mutations in the major human skeletal muscle chloride channel gene (CLCN1) leading to myotonia. *Am J Hum Genet* 1995; **57**: 1325–34.

5 Lehmann-Horn F, Mailänder V, Heine R, *et al.* Myotonia levior is a chloride channel myotonia. *Hum Mol Genet* 1995a; **4**: 1397–1402.

6 Heine R, George AL, Pika U, *et al.* Proof of a non-functional muscle chloride channel in recessive myotonia congenita (Becker) by detection of a 4 base pair deletion. *Hum Mol Genet* 1994; **3**: 1123–8.

7 Mailänder V, Heine R, Deymeer F, *et al.* Novel chloride channel mutations and their effects on heterozygous carriers. *Am J Hum Genet* 1996; **58**: 317–24.

8 Meyer-Kleine C, Ricker K, Otto M, *et al.* A recurrent 14 bp deletion in the CLCN1 gene associated with generalized myotonia (Becker). *Hum Mol Genet* 1994; **3**: 1015–6.

9 Lerche H, Mitrovic N, Dubowitz V, *et al.* Paramyotonia congenita: The R1448P sodium channel mutation in adult human skeletal muscle. *Ann Neurol* 1996; **39**: 599–608.

10 Meyer-Kleine C, Otto M, Zoll B, *et al.* Molecular and genetic characterisation of German families with paramyotonia congenita and demonstration of founder effect in the Ravensberg families. *Hum Gen* 1994; **93**: 707–10.

11 Mitrovic N, George AL Jr, Heine R, *et al.* Potassium-aggravated myotonia. Biophysical and clinical implications of the G1306A/V/E human muscle sodium channel mutations. *J Physiol* 1995; **487**: 107–14.

12 Ptáček LJ, Tawil R, Griggs RC, *et al.* Sodium channel mutations in acetazolamide-responsive myotonia congenita, paramyotonia congenita and hyperkaelmic periodic paralyses. *Neurology* 1994b; **4**: 1500–503.

13 Ricker K, Moxley RT, Heine R, *et al.* Myotonia fluctuans, a third type of muscle sodium channel disease. *Arch Neurol* 1994; **51**: 1095–102.

14 Fontaine B, Vale Santos JM, Jurkat-Rott K, *et al.* Mapping of hypokalemic periodic paralysis (HypoPP) to chromosome 1q31-q32 by a genome-wide search in three European families. *Nat Genet* 1994; **6**: 267–72.

15 Jurkat-Rott K, Lehmann-Horn F, Elbaz A, *et al.* A calcium channel mutation causing hypokalemic periodic paralysis. *Hum Mol Genet* 1994; **3**: 1414–9.

16 Ptáček L, Tawil R, Griggs RC, *et al.* Dihydropyridine receptor mutations cause hypokalemic periodic paralyses. *Cell* 1994; **77**: 863–8.

This is based on a report originally published in *Neuromuscul Disord* 1993; **3(2)**: 162–8 and on the report of the 37th ENMC International Workshop: Paramyotonia, potassium aggravated myotonias and periodic paralyses shortly to be published with permission from Pergamon Press Ltd, Headington Hill Hall, Oxford OX3 0BW, UK.

8 Spinal Muscular Atrophy

TL Munsat *Dept of Neurology, New England Medical Center, Boston, USA*

KE Davies *Genetics Laboratory, Dept of Biochemistry, University of Oxford, Oxford, UK*

▶ Diagnostic Criteria

The gene locus for childhood spinal muscular atrophy (SMA) has been localized to the long arm of chromosome 5 (5q) and diagnostic criteria are presented below.

SMA I, II and III

Clinical criteria

Age at onset

I In SMA type I (severe form) onset is from birth to 6 months;
in SMA type II (intermediate form) onset is before the age of 18 months;
in SMA type III (mild form) onset is after the age of 18 months.

C These criteria are arbitrary and subject to overlap.

Muscle weakness

I Muscle weakness of the trunk and limbs (proximal limb muscles more than distal; lower limbs weaker than upper limbs).

I Symmetrical.

E Weakness of extra-ocular muscles, diaphragm and the myocardium, or marked facial weakness.

C Wasting is often not conspicuous in SMA type I.

Other associated features

I Fasciculations of tongue and tremor of hands.

C Tremor of the hands is frequently observed in SMA types II and III.

E Sensory disturbances.

E Central nervous system dysfunction.

E Arthrogryposis.

C In SMA type I there may be some mild limitation of abduction of the hips or extension of the knees or elbows.

E Involvement of other neurological systems or organs, i.e. hearing or vision.

Course

I In SMA types I and II there is an arrest of development of motor milestones.
Children with SMA type I are never able to sit without support.
Children with SMA type II are unable to stand or walk without aid.

I In SMA type I death is usually <2 years of age.
In SMA type II death is usually above the age of 2 years.
In SMA type III death is in adulthood.

C There will be certain patients who do not clearly fit any one category.

Laboratory criteria

Biochemistry

E SCK activity >10 times the upper limit of normal.

E Dystrophin deficiency.

E Hexosaminidase deficiency.

Electrophysiology

I Abnormal spontaneous activity, i.e. fibrillations, positive sharp waves, fasciculations.

I Increased mean duration and amplitude of motor unit action potentials.

E Reduction of motor nerve conduction velocities <70% of lower limit of normal.

E Abnormal sensory nerve action potentials.

Histopathology

I Groups of atrophic fibres of both types.
Hypertrophic fibres of type I.
Type grouping (chronic cases).

'Variants' of Infantile SMA (J Ignatius)

Several patients have been described in the literature designated as infantile SMA, but with associated 'atypical' features such as cerebellar hypoplasia, pontocerebellar or cerebello-thalamospinal degeneration, multiple long bone fractures at birth, diaphragmatic paralysis with early respiratory failure and congenital heart defects. Most of these patients also had arthrogryposis. It is unclear as to whether these patients represent separate clinical entities.

Anterior horn cell disease with pontocerebellar hypoplasia

This condition might be mistaken for SMA type I because of the profound floppiness at birth, tongue fasciculations and findings consistent with anterior horn cell drop-out in EMG and muscle biopsy. However, unlike severe SMA, these infants are not alert and there may be signs of upper motor neuron involvement (brisk reflexes, jerky eye movements, pathological EEG). Multiple joint contractures are frequent and at post-mortem there is cerebellar atrophy and involvement of the pons, medulla and spinal cord.

Based on linkage analysis data obtained in one family this condition was not linked to 5q.

Anterior horn cell disease with congenital fractures

This entity is characterized by multiple congenital, metaphyseal or epiphyseal long bone fractures associated with large joint and digital contractures. It may include two separate conditions. In some families polyhydramnios, intrauterine growth retardation, hypomineralized bones and dysmorphic features are present.

The pedigrees are consistent with autosomal recessive inheritance. In some families the pregnancy is uneventful, birth weight is normal and dysmorphic features are not prominent. Pedigrees consistent with X-linked recessive inheritance have been published. The clinical pattern appears consistent among affected sibs which suggests that this is a separate entity.

Linkage analysis has been performed in one family[1]. This disorder also appears to be unlinked to 5q.

Anterior horn cell disease with early respiratory insufficiency

The presenting symptom is acute respiratory distress at birth or during the first weeks of life. Generalized muscle weakness may not be evident before disease onset. Distal joint contractures are common. The distribution of muscle weakness may be atypical (often bilateral wrist drop). Eventration or abnormal motion of the diaphragm is seen by X-ray/fluoroscopy. Findings on EMG, muscle biopsy and post-mortem have been similar to SMA.

Only a few familial cases have been reported, but the clinical pattern appears consistent among sibs, and it is likely that the condition is hereditary.

No DNA studies have been reported.

Anterior horn cell disease with congenital heart defects (S. Rudnik)

Congenital heart defects are common; they occur in 1% of births. Among these septal defects are the most common: the incidence of ventricular septal defect (VSD) is 2.5-5/1000 and that of atrial septal defect (ASD) 1/1000 live births. Thus a child presenting with both SMA and heart defect may represent a coincidence.

Congenital heart defect (most often ASD) associated with SMA has been proposed as a distinct entity. This association has now been observed among sibs. If carefully examined, however, these patients appear to have additional atypical features such as arthrogryposis, respiratory distress, bone fractures and, at post-mortem, arrhinencephaly or partial corpus callosum hypoplasia. Thus, some may actually belong with the entities described above. A heart defect associated with SMA should prompt a search for additional atypical features.

Linkage analysis has been performed in one family (J Melki) and no recombinants were found.

Anterior horn cell disease associated with arthrogryposis

When carefully studied, most patients described in the literature as having 'SMA and arthrogryposis' appear to represent entities described above. Arthrogryposis associated with anterior horn cell disease, but without other pathology, seems to be very rare.

These cases have almost invariably been sporadic. In some patients the disease has not been progressive and these may represent neurogenic arthrogryposis multiplex congenita. Arthrogryposis as an exclusion criterion is justified at present, especially for linkage studies and prenatal testing.

SMA of nonrecessive inheritance

At present there is no good evidence for X-chromosomal inheritance in childhood SMA. The patients described in the literature as X-linked severe SMA also had arthrogryposis and bone fractures. Several patients suffering from mild X-linked SMA ('SMA of adolescent onset with hypertrophied calf muscles') were later re-examined and defined as Becker muscular dystrophy.

Autosomal dominant inheritance cannot be excluded in some families with childhood-onset SMA. Based on segregation analysis data, some patients classified as SMA type II or SMA type III may represent new dominant mutations. There are also some rare pedigrees where a child born to a SMA patient (without a family history of the disease) has also been affected. Clinically, these patients are indistinguishable from those suffering from the autosomal recessive SMA5q. This possibility as well as the proposed genetic complexity at the SMA locus, has important implications for prenatal diagnosis, particularly as regards the milder forms of SMA.

Differential Diagnosis of SMA (V Dubowitz)

Several congenital myopathies may mimic SMA. However, SMA infants have very weak intercostals associated with relative sparing of the diaphragm. As a result they have highly characteristic thorax deformity and abdominal type of breathing which often allows diagnosis. In many myopathies there is also facial weakness. Muscle biopsy is an important tool to differentiate these conditions.

Congenital hypomyelination neuropathy may also mimic early onset severe SMA. This entity is rare and most cases have been sporadic. The muscle biopsy may show grouped atrophy like SMA. The differential diagnosis is based on nerve conduction velocities which are extremely slow (< 10 m/sec).

Hexosaminidase deficiency may rarely produce a clinical picture resembling juvenile SMA. The adult type of hexosaminidase A deficiency is very rare. Most patients have been of Ashkenazi Jewish origin. Signs of cerebellar dysfunction (particularly speech difficulties) are highly characteristic of this disorder and, in those cases with onset before 10 years of age, dysarthria has been invariably present. Cerebellar symptoms may appear years after clinical onset. The level of hexosaminidase A in serum and most tissues of these patients is very low.

▶ DNA Studies (KE Davies)

The mutation for autosomal recessive SMA has been mapped to chromosome 5q13 and there is very little, if any, evidence for genetic heterogeneity. Two major genes have been mapped to the region. The survival motor neuron (SMN) gene is present in two copies. Deletion of exons 7 and 8 within the telomeric copy of the SMN gene occurs in more than 95% of SMA patients. However, there is no correlation between this deletion and the severity of the phenotype. However, through the analysis of microsatellites in the region, type I patients appear to have more extensive deletions in 5q13 than the more mildly affected patients.

Further evidence supporting a major role for SMN in the disease process comes from the existence of point mutations and small deletions in the telomeric copy of the gene which introduces stop codons. However, deletions of SMN have been found in carriers and apparently phenotypically normal sibs of patients. It is possible that mutation in SMN is a critical event but that the clinical course of the disorders is dependent on other genes, either in 5q13 or elsewhere in the genome.

Whatever the role of SMN in the disease pathology, deletion of exons 7 and 8 of the telomeric gene are proving very important for the diagnosis of the disorder, especially of the mild forms of the disease.

A second candidate gene, the neuronal apoptosis inhibitor protein (NAIP) gene, may be a good candidate for the second gene or may be the major locus which is mutated. This gene has been shown recently to play a role in apoptosis and may thus play a crucial role in motor neuron survival. Exons of the NAIP gene are present through the region but there is only one functional copy of the gene. This maps close to the telomeric copy of SMN. NAIP is deleted in type I patients (~60%) more frequently than type II and III patients but is also deleted in 2–3% of phenotypically normal carriers.

For detailed references see Crawford[2].

References

1 Lunt PW, Mathew C, Clark S, *et al.* Can prenatal diagnosis be offered in neontally lethal spinal muscular atrophy (SMA) with arthrogryposis and fractures? *J Med Genet* 1992; **29**: 282 (abstract).

2 Crawford, TO. From enigmatic to problematic: the new molecular genetics of childhood spinal muscular atrophy. *Neurology* 1996; **46**: 335–40.

This is based on reports originally published in *Neuromuscul Disord* 1991; **1(2)**: 81, 1992; **2(5/6)**: 423–8, 1994; **4(2)**: 153–4, 1995; **5(4)**: 333–6, 1996; **6(2)**: 125–7, and 1996; **6(4)**: 296 with permission from Pergamon Press Ltd, Headington Hill Hall, Oxford OX3 0BW, UK

9 Familial Amyotrophic Lateral Sclerosis

M Swash *Dept of Neurology, The Royal London Hospital, London, UK*

CED Shaw and PN Leigh *Dept of Clinical Neurosciences, Institute of Psychiatry and King's College School of Medicine and Dentistry, London, UK*

▶ Diagnostic Criteria

The diagnosis of familial amyotrophic lateral sclerosis (FALS) must be consistent with that of the sporadic disease. The criteria for the diagnosis of amyotrophic lateral sclerosis (ALS) were agreed at a consensus conference held in 1990 in El Escorial, Spain. These criteria have since been ratified by the World Federation of Neurology Sub-Committee on Neuromuscular Disorders, and have been published in the *Journal of the Neurological Sciences* (1994)[1]. The relevance of such criteria is shown by studies of diagnostic behaviour in the UK and other countries in which striking differences emerged[2]. Since FALS is a form of ALS distinguished from the more common sporadic variant only by its familial background, the diagnostic criteria for FALS must follow those for the sporadic disease. In most series familial cases comprise 5–10% of cases of the disease[3,4].

The El Escorial criteria for diagnosis of ALS are shown in Table 1. These criteria take account of the difficulties associated with early diagnosis, or with incomplete clinical expression of the disease, by introducing different levels of certainty for the diagnosis, i.e. **definite, probable** and **possible** (see Tables 1 and 2). The criteria utilize the distribution of upper and lower motor neuron signs in the different regions of the body, in assigning the degree of diagnostic certainty, and allow EMG

Table 1. *El Escorial criteria for the diagnosis of ALS*.*

The diagnosis of ALS requires
The **presence** of:
1 LMN signs (including EMG features in clinically normal muscles)
2 UMN signs
3 progression of the disorder
Together with the **absence** of:
elecrophysiological or neuroimaging evidence of other disease processes

LMN=lower motor neuron; UMN=upper motor neuron.
*For more details see [1].

*Table 2. Subclassification of diagnostic criteria.**

Definite ALS
UMN+LMN signs in three regions** i.e. typical Charcot ALS
Probable ALS
UMN+LMN signs in two regions, with UMN signs rostral to LMN signs
Possible ALS
UMN+LMN signs in one region
or
UMN signs in two or three regions
or
LMN signs rostral to UMN signs e.g. monomelic ALS, progressive bulbar palsy, and primary lateral sclerosis
Suspected ALS
LMN in two or three regions e.g. progressive muscular atrophy, and other motor syndromes (see Table 3)

**Regions are defined as follows: brainstem, brachial, thorax and trunk, crural.
*For more details see [1].

features of lower motor neuron disturbance to be used in this description (Table 2). Certain positive features of the disease are recognized, and other features that serve to exclude the diagnosis are also noted (Table 3). In addition, a number of neurological conditions that may sometimes mimic the clinical presentation of ALS need to be recognized and, where necessary, excluded by appropriate clinical examination and investigation (Table 4).

Clinical variants of FALS

Classification of FALS syndrome is complicated by the existence of several discrete clinical syndromes, recognized with particular frequencies in certain geographic

Table 3. Clinical features that exclude or support the clinical diagnosis of ALS.

The diagnosis of ALS requires the absence *of the following clinical features:*
1 sensory signs
2 sphincter disturbances
3 visual disturbances
4 autonomic dysfunction
5 Parkinson's disease
6 Alzheimer-type dementia
7 certain 'mimic' syndromes (see Table 4)

The diagnosis of ALS is supported *by the following features:*
1 fasciculation in one or more regions
2 neurogenic changes in EMG studies
3 normal motor and sensory nerve conduction (distal motor latencies may be increased)
4 absence of conduction block

Table 4. Syndromes that may mimic ALS.

1	Monoclonal gammopathy with motor neuropathy
2	Other dys-immune LMN syndromes
3	Non-tumour endocrine syndromes
4	Lymphoma
5	Acute infections
6	Post-infection syndromes
7	Genetic enzyme defects
8	Exogenous toxic disorders
9	Physical injury
10	Vascular disorders
11	Spondylitic myelopathy
12	Radiation-induced neurogenic disorders
13	Creutzfeldt–Jakob disease and other prion disorders

locations, or among certain populations. Those recognized by the European FALS Collaborative Group are listed in Table 5. It is not known whether these syndromes are distinctive genetic disorders, or represent varying phenotypic expression of the same disorder.

Other ALS disorders, occurring in Guam[5,6] and Japan, and possibly also New Guinea[5] may have a genetic basis, but this is currently controversial[7]. Familial conditions in which anterior horn cell involvement occurs as part of a more

Table 5. Classification of familial ALS syndromes.

1 Typical ALS
   rapidly progressive forms (survival–median ~2 years)
   slowly progressive forms (survival–median 11 years)
2 A pure LMN syndrome with rapid progression
3 ALS associated with dementia of frontal lobe type
   (a disorder of conduct and personality)
4 Focal amyotrophy with UMN signs (non-progressive disorder)
5 Juvenile types, with onset <25 years of age:
   a classical ALS; slow progression with fasciculation
   b spastic paraparesis with atrophy of the legs
      fasciculation
      EMG neurogenic
      progressive
   c pseudo-bulbar palsy with spastic paraparesis
      atrophy of legs
      fasciculation not prominent
   d ALS with deafness
      Brown–Vialetto–van Laere syndrome
   e infantile onset bulbar palsy
      Fazio–Londe syndrome
      ?Worster–Drought syndrome

widespread neurological disease do not form part of the syndrome of FALS itself, but represent different disorders[8].

Spinal muscular atrophy syndromes are excluded from this classification of FALS, since they constitute a different group of disorders. Spinal muscular atrophy can sometimes be confused clinically with ALS, particularly in relation to sporadic cases of the progressive muscular atrophy variant of ALS.

The X-linked form of bulbo-spinal muscular atrophy (Kennedy's syndrome), now known to be linked on the X chromosome with the androgen gene[9], must be excluded in the diagnosis of all familial syndromes involving the lower motor neuron, particularly when the index case is sporadic and male, when there are no corticospinal tract signs, when there are no affected female members of the family, and when the pattern of inheritance is suggestive of X-linkage.

Similarly, whenever possible, a prion disorder must be excluded in all patients with ALS associated with dementia of the frontal type[10] or with other atypical features, e.g. extrapyramidal rigidity[11].

The clinical criteria for the diagnosis of FALS set out here are essentially intuitive, representing a consensus achieved by discussion among two groups of neurologists. They require testing by practical application and, more objectively, by an analysis such as that used by Li *et al.*[2] in their study of the consistency of diagnosis of sporadic ALS in three countries.

▶ DNA Studies (M Swash)

Since the meeting report on FALS, there have been advances in the genetics of FALS. Siddique, with colleagues, noted that FALS was expressed as an autosomal disorder, indistinguishable clinically from the commoner sporadic form of the disease[12,13]. The FALS locus was mapped in a small subset of informative families to chromosome 21q22.1[14]. Seven of 11 families tested showed this locus, and linkage to this region was excluded in three of the remaining families. It was recognized that this locus was close to that for the Cu, Zn superoxide dismutase gene (SOD-1) on chromosome 21. Subsequent studies have co-localized the locus with that for SOD-1 in these affected families, and have demonstrated mutations in exons 1, 2, 3 and 5 respectively in some of these families[15,16]. There are five exons in the SOD-1 gene. SOD-1 activity in individuals with SOD-1 gene mutations varies from about 30% to normal. These data add an intriguing dimension to the notion that neurodegeneration in ALS might be due, at least in part, to an abnormality in the ability of susceptible motorneuron pools to handle free radicals[17,18]. The evidence for this mechanism of pathogenesis in ALS is increasingly persuasive, but does not take account of those families in which a mutation in the SOD-1 gene has been excluded, and does not yet provide an entirely plausible explanation for sporadic cases. Nonetheless, the discovery of the role of mutations in the SOD-1 gene in some familial cases illustrates the power of genetic analysis in revealing hitherto unsuspected metabolic abnormalities in progressive degenerative disorders.

References

1 El Escorial World Federation of Neurology criteria for the diagnosis of ALS. *J Neurol Sci* 1994, 124 (Suppl): 96–107.

2 Li T-M, Swash M, Alberman A, Day SJ. Diagnosis of motor neuron disease in three countries. *J Neurol Neurosurg Psychiatry* 1991; **54**: 980–3.

3 Li T-M, Alberman E, Swash M. Comparison of sporadic and familial disease amongst 580 cases of motor neuron disease. *J Neurol Neurosurg Psychiatry* 1988; 51: 778–84.

4 Williams DB, Floate DA, Leicester J. Familial motor neurone disease: differing patterns in large pedigrees. *J Neurol Sci* 1988; **86**: 215–30.

5 Gajdusek DC. Environmental factors provoking physiological changes which induce motor neuron disease and early neuronal aging in high incidence foci in the Western Pacific. In: Rose FC, ed. *Research progress in motor neuron disease.* Pitman: London, 1984: 44–69.

6 Garruto RM, Yanagihara R, Gajdusek DC. Disappearance of high incidence amyotrophic lateral sclerosis and Parkinson-dementia on Guam. *Neurology* 1985; 35: 193–8.

7 Duncan MW. Role of the Cycad neurotoxin BMAA in the amyotrophic lateral sclerosis–Parkinsonism–dementia complex of the Western Pacific. In: Rowland LP, ed. *Amyotrophic lateral sclerosis and other motor neuron diseases,* Advances in Neurology, Vol. 56. Raven Press: New York, 1991: 301–10.

8 Schwartz MS, Swash M. Motor neuron disease. In: Swash M, Oxbury J, eds. *Clinical neurology.* Churchill Livingstone: Edinburgh, 1991: 1356–66.

9 La Spada AR, Wilson EM, Lubahn DB, Harding AE, Fischbeck KH. Androgen receptor gene mutation in X-linked spinal and bulbar atrophy. *Nature* 1991; **352**: 77–9.

10 Neary D, Snowden JS, Mann DMA, Northen P, Goulding PJ, MacDermott N. Frontal lobe dementia and motor neuron disease. *J Neurol Neurosurg Psychiatry* 1990; **53**: 23–32.

11 Mitsuyama Y. Presenile dementia with motor neuron disease in Japan; clinicopathological review of 26 cases. *J Neurol Neurosurg Psychiatry* 1984; **47**: 953–9.

12 Siddique T, Pericak-Vance MA, Brooks BR, *et al.* Linkage analysis in familial amyotrophic lateral sclerosis. *Neurology* 1989; **39**: 919–25.

13 Mulder DW, Kurland LT, Offord KP, Beard M. Familial adult motor neuron disease: amyotrophic lateral sclerosis. *Neurology* 1986; **36**: 511–7.

14 Siddique T, Figlewicz DA, Pericak-Vance MA, *et al.* Linkage of a gene causing familial amyotrophic lateral sclerosis to chromosome 21 and evidence of genetic-locus heterogeneity. *NEJM* 1991; **324**: 1381–4.

15 Rosen DR, Siddique T, Patterson D, *et al.* Mutations in Cu/Zn superoxide dismutase gene are associated with familial amyotrophic lateral sclerosis. *Nature* 1993; **362**: 59–62.

16 Deng H-X, Hentati A, Tainer JA, *et al.* Amyotrophic lateral sclerosis and structural defects in Cu, Zn superoxide dismutase. *Science* 1993; **261**: 1047–51.

17 Hallewell RA, Gutteridge JMC. Oxygen radicals and the nervous system. *Trends in Neurosciences* 1985; **8**: 22–6.

18 Brown RH. Amyotrophic lateral sclerosis: recent insights from genetics and transgenic mice. *Cell* 1995; **80**: 687–92.

This is partly based on a report originally published in *Neuromuscul Disord* 1992; **2(1)**: 7–9 with permission from Pergamon Press Ltd, Headington Hill Hall, Oxford OX3 0BW, UK

10 Hereditary Motor and Sensory Neuropathy or Charcot–Marie–Tooth Disease Types IA and IB

M de Visser *Dept of Neurology, Academic Medical Centre, Amsterdam, The Netherlands*

C van Broeckhoven and E Nelis *Neurogenetics Laboratory, Flemish Institute for Biotechnology, Born-Bunge Foundation, University of Antwerp, Dept of Biochemistry, Antwerp, Belgium*

▶ Diagnostic Criteria

Charcot–Marie–Tooth (CMT) disease is a clinically and genetically heterogeneous peripheral neuropathy characterized by wasting and weakness of the distal limb muscles. CMT I, the demyelinating form, and CMT II, the axonal form, are the most common types with an estimated prevalence of at least 1 in 10 000. Inheritance pattern is autosomal dominant in the majority of patients.

Positional cloning has shown that CTM I is genetically heterogeneous with at least three loci. The major autosomal dominant subtype CMT IA is linked to chromosome 17p11.2. A less frequent autosomal dominant subtype, CMT IB, is linked to chromosome 1q22-q23, and a third also autosomal dominant subtype, CMT IC, is not linked to either of these loci and as yet unassigned.

In the majority of CMT IA patients, either familial or sporadic, the disease is associated with a tandem DNA duplication of 1.5 Mb. This duplication can be detected by density differences in the alleles or by the presence of three alleles of polymorphic DNA probes or microsatellite markers, or by a duplication junction fragment with pulsed field gel electrophoresis technology. Almost all patients, independent of their ethnic origin, have the same sized duplication. The collaborative duplication screening of the European Consortium on CMT I resulted in a duplication frequency of 70.7%. The duplication was found to contain the human homologue of the peripheral myelin protein-22 gene (PMP-22). PMP-22 is not altered by the duplication and shows a dosage effect in CMT IA patients. In nonduplicated CMT IA patients point mutations in PMP-22 confirmed the direct role of the gene in the CMT IA disease process.

In CMT IB mutations in the myelin protein zero gene (MPZ) appeared to co-segregate with the disease.

In May 1991, the ENMC Consortium established diagnostic criteria for autosomal dominant CMT I. These criteria were meant to serve only for research purposes, and in particular for linkage analysis. However, a diagnosis of autosomal dominant CMT I can now be accurately made by detection of the duplication or by identification of a point mutation in either the PMP-22 or MPZ gene. Therefore, we have amended the diagnostic criteria on CMT IA and CMT IB accordingly by adding DNA analysis as an inclusion criterion. Furthermore, over the years genotype–phenotype correlations have extended our knowledge of the clinical picture of CMT I. Some patients who once had been diagnosed as suffering from Dejerine–Sottas disease were found to have a PMP-22 or MPZ point mutation.

Linkage studies in other subtypes of CMT have yielded loci on chromosome 8q for one form of **autosomal recessive CMT I** (with basal lamina onion bulbs) and on chromosomes 1p and 3q, respectively for two subtypes of the **autosomal dominantly inherited CMT II**. An **X-linked dominant form of CMT** with demyelinating and neuronal characteristics also manifests with distal muscle wasting and weakness. Males usually have more pronounced clinical features than females. After assignment of the locus to Xq13.1, mutations in the gene encoding connexin 32 (Cx32), a gap junction protein were found in most CMTX patients.

Hereditary neuropathy with liability to pressure palsies (HNPP) is hallmarked by periodic episodes of weakness or numbness often due to minor compression or trauma to peripheral nerves. In some patients HNPP may mimic CMT. The disease which is inherited as an autosomal dominant trait is usually associated with a deletion in chromosome 17p11.2 encompassing the same markers that are duplicated in CMT IA. A few HNPP patients have point mutations in PMP-22.

An overview of the duplication/deletion and mutation screening techniques and an estimation of the mutation frequencies in CMT I and HNPP patients is found in Nelis *et al.*[1].

It is of note that as yet no attempts have been undertaken to establish diagnostic criteria for the above mentioned subtypes of CMT.

The following criteria for inclusion (I) and exclusion (E) of the diagnosis are only applicable to the autosomal dominant forms of CMT I in which the duplication or a point mutation in either the PMP-22 or MPZ gene is present, i.e., CMT IA and CMT IB, (C) refers to comments.

Clinical criteria

Family history

I Autosomal dominant inheritance

C Isolated cases as a result of a *de novo* duplication are found in a proportion of the patients.

Age at onset

I Usually in the first two decades of life.

C Congenital onset with floppiness is very rare.

Muscle wasting and weakness

I Muscle wasting and weakness of predominantly the distal part of the lower limbs.

I Symmetrical.

C Later, wasting and weakness of the intrinsic hand muscles and the distal part of the medial vastus muscle and other parts of the quadriceps muscle may develop.

Other associated features or diseases

C Impaired sensation is frequently observed but is not an obligatory feature.

E Arthrogryposis with the exception of talipes or pes cavus.

C Scoliosis and nerve hypertrophy are present in a proportion of the patients.

E CNS involvement.

C The presence of brisk reflexes should militate against the diagnosis. Some patients may have extensor plantar responses. There may be tremor or slight limb ataxia.

E Other major organ involvement (vision, hearing, cardiac).

C There may be abnormalities of visual or auditory evoked responses but no overt clinical evidence of involvement of the optic or auditory nerves.

E Impairment of oculomotor and bulbar function; marked facial weakness.

E Myotonic dystrophy.

Course and severity

I Slowly progressive or stationary over long periods of time.

C At any age there is a wide range of severity.

C Some patients are asymptomatic and are found to have pes cavus and/or areflexia on examination. Rarely, proximal muscles may become involved leading to wheelchair dependence or respiratory insufficiency.

Laboratory criteria

Electrophysiology

I Median nerve motor conduction velocity (MCV) $\leqslant$38 m/sec. Absence or marked decrease of sensory nerve action potentials (SNAPs) in the lower limbs.

C An occasional patient may have, at some time in the course of the disease, a median nerve MCV up to 40–45 m/sec. If so, the contralateral median and/or ulnar nerve should be investigated.

C Electromyography may show signs of denervation and reinnervation.

Molecular genetics

I Duplication of 1.5 Mb (rarely smaller) on 17p11.2 or, in non-duplicated patients point mutations in the myelin gene PMP-22 designates CMT IA.

I In non-duplicated patients point mutations in the myelin gene MPZ designates CMT IB.

Sensory nerve biopsy

(Usually sural nerve although a fibular nerve may sometimes be sampled.)

I Characteristic features are the following:
Marked reduction of density and total number of large and small myelinated fibres
Segmental demyelination and remyelination.
An increase in total transverse fascicular area
Onion bulbs
Axonal changes are usually not prominent.

C With the introduction of DNA-analysis as a diagnostic tool nerve biopsies should no longer be used for establishing the diagnosis.

Reference

1 Nelis E, Van Broeckhoven C. Estimation of the mutation frequencies in CMT I and HNPP: a European collaborative study. *Eur J Hum Genet* 1996; **4**: 25–33.

This is partly based on a report originally published in *Neuromuscul Disord* 1993; **3(1)**: 77–9 with permission from Pergamon Press Ltd, Headington Hill Hall, Oxford OX3 0BW, UK

11

Chronic Inflammatory Neuropathies

H Franssen *Dept of Clinical Neurophysiology, University Hospital Utrecht, The Netherlands*
M Vermeulen *Dept of Neurology, Academic Medical Centre, Amsterdam, The Netherlands*
FGI Jennekens *Dutch Neuromuscular Research Support Centre, Baarn, The Netherlands*

▶ Introduction

Research criteria for chronic inflammatory demyelinating polyneuropathy (CIDP) were first proposed and published by an Ad Hoc Subcommittee of the American Academy of Neurology in 1991[1]. Since then several important developments have taken place. Multifocal motor neuropathy (MMN) was recognized as related to CIDP, but is different in several respects. Definition and recognition of electrophysiological phenomena, as for example 'conduction block' and 'temporal dispersion' was improved. Therefore it became desirable to adapt the criteria introduced in 1991.

Recent reports suggest that the group of chronic inflammatory neuropathy consists of several entities. Among these are chronic inflammatory sensory neuropathy and chronic inflammatory (or autoimmune) axonal neuropathy. The present criteria concern only CIDP and MMN. They were agreed upon at two consensus workshops organized by the Dutch Neuromuscular Research Support Centre in October 1995 and April 1996.

▶ Diagnostic Criteria for CIDP

Elements

1 CIDP may occur at all ages (in all decades)[2,3].
2 CIDP is a chronic disease. It does not reach nadir until 8 weeks after onset. The course is progressive, stepwise progressive or relapsing[2,3].
3 The clinical signs involve muscle weakness and/or sensory disturbances. Motor or sensory abnormalities are absent in some cases[2,3].
4 The distribution of the clinical signs is (approximately) symmetrical. The first signs appear distal at the limbs, in some cases initially or predominantly at the

upper limbs[3,4]. Marked weakness of the lower limbs with approximately normal muscle power at the upper limbs is unusual. Weakness of neck extensors presenting as a 'dropped head syndrome' has been described[5].

5 Cranial nerves (nerves innervating the extra-ocular muscles and facial and hypoglossus nerves) may be involved[2,3].

6 Sensory disturbances concern predominantly large sensory nerve fibre modalities. Disturbances due to small sensory nerve fibre involvement and autonomic disturbances are rare[2].

7 Tendon reflexes are reduced or absent in most cases[2,4].

8 At some time during the course of the disease postural tremor may become apparent[2,3].

9 There may be papilloedema[2,3].

10 Nerve conduction of motor nerve fibres is abnormal and compatible with demyelination[1,6]. Abnormalities are not present to the same degree in all (mixed) nerves. Details on the electrophysiological methods are provided in the Addendum page 57.

Motor conduction velocity (MCV) including F-waves is examined in four nerves (ulnar, median, peroneal, tibial) on one side of the body. Sensory conduction on distal stimulation is examined in the median, ulnar, and sural nerves on the same side as motor conduction. Three of the following four items (at least one in an upper limb) should be present:

a Motor conduction velocity (MCV) less than 75% of the lower limit of normal in at least two nerves.
(Lower limits of normal MCV are generally considered to be 50 m/sec in upper limb nerves and 40 m/sec in lower limb nerves. Values compatible with demyelination are therefore 38 m/sec and 30 m/sec or less).

b Definite or possible conduction block in at least one nerve segment.

c Distal motor latency (DML) more than 130% of the upper limit of normal in at least two nerves.

d Absence of F-wave, or shortest F-wave latency more than 130% of the upper limit of normal, in at least one nerve.

11 The protein content of the cerebrospinal fluid (CSF) is raised. It is raised in 90–95% of all cases to more than 0.5 g/l and often to more than 1 g/l[2]. The CSF cell count is less than 30×10^6/l; this may be higher in HIV patients with CIDP.

12 A sural nerve biopsy may reveal active demyelination and mononuclear inflammatory cell infiltrates[7].

13 MRI reveals white matter lesions in a minority of the cases[8].

14 CIDP may be associated with: systemic lupus erythematosus, Hodgkin's disease, ulcerative colitis, multiple sclerosis, myasthenia gravis, psoriasis, diabetes mellitus, hyperthyroidism, and HIV[2,3]. In patients with MGUS (monoclonal gammopathy of unknown significance) a peripheral neuropathy fulfilling the criteria of CIDP may occur.

15 Other neuropathies to be excluded include:

a Pure sensory neuropathies including ganglioneuritis and mixed neuropathies with predominant loss of small sensory nerve fibre modalities.

b Axonal neuropathies.

c Charcot–Marie–Tooth (CMT) neuropathies (CMT neuropathies differ from CIDP in symptoms, electrophysiological signs, course, family history).

d Meningeal carcinomatosis or lymphomatosis (often cranial nerve involvement and conus/cauda syndrome, diagnosis by CSF cytology).

e Other neuropathies with relapsing course (hereditary neuropathy with liability to pressure palsies, Refsum disease (this neuropathy is associated with night blindness and often with deafness, the phytanic acid level in serum is raised), Tangier disease (disturbance predominantly of small sensory nerve fibre qualities, conduction velocity is only moderately reduced).
f Other demyelinating neuropathies, e.g. paraproteinaemic neuropathies and neuropathies in rare hereditary disorders as metachromatic leucodystrophy and Krabbe disease.
g Infectious diseases of the peripheral nervous system, e.g. Lyme neuroborreliosis, (pleocytosis, raised serum antibody titres).
h Iatrogenic, toxic and metabolic neuropathies.

Assessment

From the above it is clear that CIDP can be diagnosed when patients with the clinical features of a chronic sensory-motor polyneuropathy, and a raised protein content of the cerebrospinal fluid, reveal evidence of demyelination at electrophysiological investigation, and when other possible causes have been ruled out. The diagnosis is less certain when one of these four features is weak or absent. In figures:

The diagnosis is **definite**, when:
a 2, 3, 4, 7, 10 and 11 are all present and findings exclude 15
b the presence of 6 and/or 12 concurs with the diagnosis but is not a requirement
c the presence of 5, 8, 9, 13, 14 is compatible with the diagnosis

The diagnosis is **probable**, when:
a 2, 3, 4, 7 and 11 are all present, 10 is partly present (less than three of the specified items are present) and findings exclude 15
b the presence of 6 and/or 12 is in support of the diagnosis
c the presence of 5, 8, 9, 13, 14 is compatible with the diagnosis

The diagnosis is **possible**, when:
a 2, 3, 4, 7, 11 are all present and findings exclude to 15
b the presence of 6 is in support of the diagnosis
c the presence of 5, 8, 9 and 14 is reason to consider the diagnosis

▶ Diagnostic Criteria for MMN

Elements

1 MMN is a chronic disease. Nadir is not reached until 8 weeks after onset, the course of the disease is progressive, or stepwise progressive, or undulating over many months or years[9,10].
2 Muscle weakness, muscle atrophy, fasciculations and muscle cramps are the main clinical signs. Muscle weakness may be present in non-atrophic muscles. Slight sensory disturbances do not rule out the diagnosis. Cranial nerves are rarely involved[9,10].
3 Signs of the disease are initially asymmetric and remain asymmetric in most patients[9,10].

4 The disease usually begins at the upper limbs, predominantly distal.[9,10].

5 Tendon reflexes in affected limbs are decreased or absent. Generalized absence of reflexes may occur[9,10].

6 Motor conduction block is present. The changes in MCV are compatible with multifocal asymmetric demyelination[9,10]. Sensory conduction is usually normal, also in segments with motor conduction block. Slight sensory conduction abnormalities are however compatible with the diagnosis[9,10]. Electromyography reveals spontaneous muscle fibre activity and polyphasic or giant motor unit potentials, in an asymmetric distribution. Critera for motor conduction block and details of the electrophysiological methods are discussed in the Addendum.

Motor nerve conduction including F-waves with recording from hand and/or foot muscles should be examined in the median, ulnar and peroneal nerves on both sides. When no evidence of conduction block can be obtained, additional nerves should be studied, especially nerves to weak non-atrophic lower or upper arm muscles. These nerves include the median, musculocutaneous, axillary and tibial nerves. Sensory conduction on distal stimulation is examined in median, ulnar, and sural nerves at one side of the body and in nerve segments in which conduction block is present.

7 The protein content of the cerebrospinal fluid is in most cases not raised and if so only slightly (less than 1 g/l)[9,10].

8 Diseases as mentioned in point 15 of the CIDP elements are excluded.

9 When the diagnosis is possible but not highly probable the presence of a raised serum titre of anti-GM-1 antibodies will increase the likelihood of the diagnosis (from an *a priori* chance of 20–60% to 50–85%)[11].

Assessment

The elements show that the diagnosis depends on the combination of a typical clinical picture and the presence of motor conduction block. In some cases the electrophysiological findings do not fully meet the criteria for definite motor conduction block; the diagnosis is still likely in these cases still likely but is no longer definite. In other cases extensive electrophysiological examination does not provide any evidence for conduction block, but this does not imply that it is excluded. The diagnosis is still possible when the clinical features are typical and evidence of demyelination is present[12].

The diagnosis is **definite** when:

a 1, 2, 3, 6 and 8 are all present

b There is "definite conduction block" with or without additional evidence of demyelination

c 4, 5, 7 and 9 concur with the diagnosis, but may be absent.

The diagnosis is **probable** when:

a 1, 2, 3 and 8 are present and when 6 is present partially

b there is "possible conduction block" with or without further evidence of demyelination

c 4, 5, 7 and 9 are in support of the diagnosis.

The diagnosis is **possible** when:

a 1, 2, 3, and 8 are present and when 6 includes evidence of demyelination but not of conduction block

b 4, 5, 7 and 9 are in support of the diagnosis.

Addendum to the electrophysiological examination of the chronic inflammatory demyelinating neuropathies

Recording and stimulation sites for motor conduction studies

Nerve	Recording site	Stimulation sites
Median	M. abductor pollicis brevis	Wrist, elbow, axilla, Erb's point
Median	M. flexor carpi radialis	Elbow, axilla, Erb's point
Ulnar	M. abductor dig. V	Wrist, 5 cm distal to elbow, 5 cm proximal to elbow, axilla, Erb's point
Musculocutaneous	M. biceps brachii	Axilla, Erb's point
Axillary	M. deltoideus	Axilla, Erb's point
Peroneal	M. extensor dig brevis	Ankle, 5 cm distal to fibular head, popliteal fossa
Tibial	M. abductor hallucis brevis	Ankle, popliteal fossa

The results of stimulation at Erb's point should be interpreted with caution as stimulation may not be supramaximal.

Slowing of conduction and demyelination

It has been reasonably established that a decrease of maximal conduction velocity or an increase of DML beyond a certain value suggests demyelination. Conduction velocity and histology of the sural nerve and other nerves have been compared in CMT neuropathy types I and II, experimental allergic neuritis and controls. Values for MCV, DML and F-wave latency have thus been obtained that are compatible with demyelination. On this basis values for MCV lower than 75% of the lower limit of normal and for DML or shortest F-wave latency of more than 130% of the upper limit of normal are considered to be indicative of demyelination[1]. Conclusions about the shortest F-wave latency should be based on findings at 16–20 responses at distal stimulation. F-wave findings should only be included as an item suggesting demyelination if DML and MCV in the same nerve do not reach values compatible with demyelination. Under these latter conditions, absence of F-waves is considered compatible with demyelination.

Conduction block

The detection of (partial) motor conduction block rests upon a reduction in the compound muscle action potential (CMAP) amplitude or area at proximal versus distal stimulation of a nerve segment. There are no generally accepted criteria for (partial) motor conduction block. A major problem is that demyelination may result in increased differences between conduction times of action potentials in individual nerve fibres. This 'temporal dispersion' also causes reduction in CMAP amplitude or area and an increase in CMAP duration on proximal versus distal stimulation, especially when conduction distance is large. It is nevertheless likely that an area reduction of more than 50% regardless of distance and duration increase is due to conduction block in at least some nerve fibres[13]. This is also true for an amplitude and area reduction of at least 30% over a short distance as found by inching. The criterion suggested by Feasby *et al.* (1985) (amplitude reduction of at least 20%) as used in the Research Criteria of the American Academy of Neurology (1991) is probably too liberal and may yield false positive results[1,14]. On the basis of these considerations criteria for conduction block were defined.

Definite conduction block: reduction in CMAP area of at least 50%, independent of conduction distance, or a reduction in CMAP amplitude and area of at least 30% over a short distance, detected by inching.

Possible conduction block: a reduction in CMAP amplitude of at least 30% for upper limb nerves and 40% for lower limb nerves[15].

Nerve anastomosis should be excluded as possible cause for CMAP reduction.

Minimal CMAP amplitudes

Values for MCV, DML and F-wave should be obtained from nerves which induce at distal stimulation a CMAP with an amplitude of at least 0.5 mV (from the baseline to the peak of negative deflection).

For the diagnosis of conduction block to be acceptable the amplitude of the negative deflection the CMP should be at least 1 mV.

Entrapment sites

Values of MCV, DML compatible with demyelination or conduction block at common entrapment sites (median nerve at the carpal tunnel, ulnar nerve at the elbow, peroneal nerve at the fibular head) should be considered as due to entrapment (and not to CIDP or MMN) unless sensory conduction at these sites is normal.

Skin temperature

When the skin temperature at the level of ankle or wrist is below 32 °C, the lower leg or the lower arm should be warmed in water to 37 °C for a period of at least 20 minutes[16]. Warming by an infrared heater is insufficient.

The application of correction factors to correct for low temperature is not justified as the relation between temperature and conduction is altered in demyelinating neuropathy[17]. Conduction block may be apparent only at a temperature in the high physiological range and may be missed at lower temperatures[17].

References

1 Ad Hoc Subcommittee of the American Academy of Neurology AIDS Task Force: Research criteria for diagnosis of chronic inflammatory demyelinating polyneuropathy. *Neurology* 1991; 41: 617–8.

2 Dyck PJ, Prineas J, Pollard J. Chronic inflammatory demyelinating polyradiculoneuropathy. In: Dyck PJ, Thomas PK, Griffin JW, Low PA, Poduslo JF ed. *Peripheral neuropathy*, Vol 2, 3rd edn. Philadelphia: WB Saunders, 1993: 1498–517.

3 McCombe PA, Pollard JD, McLeod JG. Chronic inflammatory demylinating polyradiculoneuropathy. A clinical and electrophysiological study of 92 cases. *Brain* 1987; **10**: 1617–30.

4 Vermeulen M, van Doorn PA, Brand A, *et al.* Intravenous immunoglobulin treatment in patients with chronic inflammatory demyelinating polyneuropathy: a double blind placebo controlled study. *J Neurol Neurosurg Psychiatry* 1993; **56**: 36–9.

5 Hoffman D, Gutmann L. The dropped head syndrome with chronic inflammatory demyelinating polyneuropathy. *Muscle Nerve* 1994; **17**: 808–10.

6 Bromberg MB. Comparison of electrodiagnostic criteria for primary demyelination in chronic polyneuropathy. *Muscle Nerve* 1991; **14**: 968–76.

7 Prineas JW. Pathology of inflammatory demyelinating neuropathies. In: JG McLeod (Ed), *Inflammatory neuropathies, Baillière's Clinical Neurology*, London: Baillière Tindall, 1994; **43**: 1–24.

8 Feasby TE, Hahn AF, Koopman RN, *et al.* Central lesions in chronic inflammatory demyelinating polyneuropathy. *Neurology* 1990; **40**: 476–8.

9 Parry GJ. Motor neuropathy with multifocal conduction block. In: Dyck PJ, Thomas PK, Griffin JW, Low PA, Poduslo JF, eds. *Peripheral neuropathy*, Vol 2, 3rd edn. Philadelphia: WB Saunders, 1993; 1518–24.

10 Parry GJ. AAEM Case report 30: Multifocal motor neuropathy. *Muscle Nerve* 1996; **19**: 269–76.

11 van Schaik IN, Bossuyt PMM, Brand A, *et al.* Diagnostic value of GM_1 antibodies in motor neuron disorders and neuropathies. *Neurology* 1995; **45**: 1570–7.

12 Pakiam A, Parry G. Multifocal motor neuropathy without evidence of conduction block. *Neurology* 1996; **46**: A 234.

13 Rhee EK, England JD, Sumner AJ. A computer simulation of conduction block: effects produced by actual block versus interphase cancellation. *Ann Neurol* 1990; **28**: 146–56.

14 Feasby T, Brown WF, Gilbert JJ, *et al.* The pathological basis of conduction block in human neuropathies. *J Neurol Neurosurg Psychiatry* 1985; **48**: 239–44.

15 Albers JW, Donofrio PD, McGonagle TK. Sequential electrodiagnostic abnormalities in acute inflammatory demyelinating polyradiculoneuropathy. *Muscle Nerve* 1985; **8**: 528–39.

16 Franssen H, Wieneke GH. Nerve conduction and temperature: necessary warming time. *Muscle Nerve* 1994; **17**: 336–44.

17 Franssen H, Wienke GH, Notermans NC, *et al.* Temperature dependent conduction block in peripheral neuropathy. *Neuro Orthopedics* 1995; **17/18**: 72–82.

12

Distal Myopathies

Hannu Somer *Dept of Neurology, University of Helsinki, Helsinki, Finland*

▶ Diagnostic Criteria

Distal myopathies comprise a group of disorders which cause distal muscle weakness without clinically significant involvement of proximal, facial or trunk muscles. Clinical examination reveals no signs of neurogenic involvement. Nerve conduction velocities are normal and electromyographic studies are compatible with myopathy without additional findings, such as myotonic discharges. SCK activity may be mildly elevated, except for in one variety where it is remarkably elevated to a level seen in generalized muscular dystrophies.

Muscle biopsy shows typical signs of myopathy such as variation in fibre size, central nuclei and increased connective tissue at an early stage. Later on more marked alterations appear. Rimmed vacuoles are seen frequently in some distal myopathies.

Central cores, nemaline bodies, inclusion bodies, glycogen or lipid accumulations seen in some patients with distal muscle weakness, are excluded from this group and suggest other diagnostic entities.

Diagnosis and classification of distal myopathies is based on clinical, genetic and morphological criteria. The following clinical phenotypes can currently be defined.

▶ Late adult onset myopathy with onset in hands[1] (Welander)

This is the most common form of the distal myopathies, by 1951 249 Swedish patients had been described[1]. The pattern of inheritance is autosomal dominant with penetrance of about 70 to 80%. The initial symptoms are clumsiness of small precise hand movements and difficulties in extension of fingers. Distal leg muscle weakness develops later on causing difficulties in walking and inability to stand on heels. Clinical course is slowly progressive. Many patients complain of coldness of hands and feet, but sensation is normal. SCK may be mildly elevated. Muscle imaging (CT or MRI) shows involvement of lower leg muscles both in the anterior and posterior compartments. Muscle biopsy from anterior tibial muscle shows myopathic changes and occasional vacuolation. Electromyography is 'myopathic' in the early stages but 'neurogenic' changes have been described especially in patients with severe muscle weakness[2].

Late adult onset myopathy with onset in legs[3,4] (Markesbery and Griggs; Udd).

The original description comes from the United States[3]. Subsequently, a similar phenotype has been described in Finland[4], where more than 100 patients have now been discovered. Muscle weakness appears usually after the age of 35 years and is confined to lower leg muscles, especially to tibial anterior muscles. The American family also developed weakness of the intrinsic hand muscles and some proximal muscle weakness. The disease is inherited in an autosomal dominant fashion.

SCK may be mildly elevated. Electromyographic changes are myopathic. These, as well as abnormal findings in muscle imaging (CT or MRI), are confined mainly to anterior tibial muscles, although mild abnormalities may also be detected elsewhere. Histopathological changes are myopathic with a spectrum from mild changes to severe end stage changes. Rimmed vacuoles may be present.

Early adult onset myopathy with onset in posterior compartment of lower legs[5] (Miyoshi).

The initial symptoms include difficulty in climbing stairs or running. Patients can not hop on one leg. Muscle weakness is most pronounced in the gastrocnemius muscle. Intrinsic foot muscles and muscles of the anterior compartment may also be involved as the disease progresses. Some patients have muscle weakness in their hand muscles. Electromyographic studies show myopathic findings. Muscle imaging studies show pronounced lesions in the posterior compartment muscles in the lower legs. SCK is elevated 10 to 100-fold being much higher than in other distal myopathies. Muscle biopsy shows severe myopathic changes in biopsies from proximal muscles. The disease is inherited in an autosomal recessive fashion[5]. Several families have been reported in Japan, United States, Tunisia and from various European countries[6].

Early adult onset myopathy with onset in anterior compartment of lower legs[7] (Nonaka).

The initial symptom is distal muscle weakness in the anterior compartment of lower legs presenting with foot drop. Later, posterior compartment muscles may become involved, but intrinsic foot muscles are usually spared. SCK is only mildly elevated. Numerous rimmed vacuoles are typical of this entity. The disease is inherited in an autosomal recessive fashion[7].

Other possible entities

In an Australian family[8] selective weakness of the toes and flexors appeared before the age of 25 years, followed by progressive weakness of finger extensors. Certain proximal muscle groups were mildly affected. The disease was inherited in an autosomal dominant fashion. Some families have been described with distal myopathy appearing in adulthood and associated with desmin storage and autophagocytosis[9,10]. The clinical course is variable, some showing rapid progression. Progression may extend to bulbar, respiratory and facial muscles. Cardiomyopathy with various conduction defects is common.

▶ DNA Studies

In the Australian family[8] positive linkage was obtained with 14 out of 15 markers tested on chromosome 14. Maximum two point lod scores of 2.60 at recombination fraction (0)=0.00 were obtained for two markers MYH7 and D14S64 – the family structure precludes a two-point lod score of 3 or greater. Recombinations with D14S72 and D14S49 indicate that this distal myopathy locus should lie between these markers.

The Miyoshi myopathy has been recently localized to chromosome 2p12–14 locus D2S291 (Z max=15.3 at 0 — =0). The results are based on patient material obtained from Japan, Tunisia and the United States[11].

References

1 Welander L. Myopathia distalis tarda hereditaria: 249 examined cases in 72 pedigrees. *Acta Med Scand* 1951; **141**: 1–124.

2 Borg K, Åhlberg G, Borg J, *et al.* Welander's distal myopathy: clinical, neurophysiological and muscle biopsy observations in young and middle aged adults with early symptoms. *J Neurol Neurosurg Psychiatry* 1991; **54**: 494–8.

3 Markesbery WR, Griggs RC, Leach RP, *et al.* Late onset hereditary distal myopathy. *Neurology* 1974; **23**: 127–34.

4 Udd B, Partanen J, Halonen P, *et al.* Tibial muscular dystrophy. Late adult onset distal myopathy in 66 Finnish patients. *Arch Neurol* 1993; **50**: 604–8.

5 Miyoshi K, Kawai H, Iwasa M, *et al.* Autosomal recessive distal muscular dystrophy as a new type of muscular dystrophy: seventeen cases in eight families, including an autopsied case. *Brain* 1986; **109**: 31–54.

6 Kuhn E, Schröder JM. Autosomal recessively inherited distal myopathy. A new type of distal myopathy. *J Neurol* 1981; **226**: 181–5.

7 Nonaka I, Sunohara N, Satoyoshi E. Familial distal myopathy with rimmed vacuole and lamellar (myeloid) body formation. *J Neurol Sci* 1981; **51**: 141–55.

8 Laing NG, Laing BA, Meredith C, *et al.* Autosomal dominant distal myopathy: linkage to chromosome 14. *Am J Hum Genet* 1995; **56**: 422–7.

9 Edström L, Thornell LE, Eriksson A. A new type of hereditary distal myopathy with characteristic sarcoplasmic bodies and intermediate (skeletin) filaments. *J Neurol Sci* 1990; **47**: 171–90.

10 Horowitz SH, Schmalbruch H. Autosomal dominant distal myopathy with desmin storage: a clinicopathological and electrophysiological study of a large kinship. *Muscle Nerve* 1994; **17**: 151–60.

11 Bejaoui K, Hirabayashi K, Hentati F, *et al.* Linkage of Miyoshi myopathy (distal autosomal recessive muscular dystrophy) locus to chromosome 2p 12–14. *Neurology* 1995; **45**: 768–72.

This is based on a report originally published in *Neuromuscul Disord* 1995; **5(3)**: 249–52 with permission from Pergamon Press Ltd, Headington Hill Hall, Oxford OX3 0BW, UK.

13 Myotubular/ Centronuclear Myopathy

C Wallgren-Pettersson *Dept of Medical Genetics, University of Helsinki, and the Folkhälsan Dept of Medical Genetics, Helsinki, Finland*

▶ Diagnostic Criteria

All forms of myotubular myopathy are extremely rare, including the usually very severe X-linked recessive form with pre- or neonatal onset (McKusick *310400), the autosomal recessive form with onset in infancy or childhood (McKusick 255200) and the relatively mild autosomal dominant form with late onset (McKusick *160150).

Consensus definitions of clinical core criteria for the X-linked form of myotubular myopathy (XMTM) include male sex, perinatal onset and severe generalized muscle hypotonia and weakness associated with ventilatory insufficiency, and often a fatal course. Additional features may include polyhydramnios, swallowing difficulties, thin ribs, contractures of the hips or knees, puffy eyelids, ophthalmoplegia and cryptorchidism. The contractures tend to be less severe than in congenital myotonic dystrophy. These boys are often long and light for both length and gestational age, with large heads. In comparison with infants with myotonic dystrophy, they seem to lack diaphragmatic elevation and upturning of the upper lip. Evidence suggesting X-linked inheritance may include miscarriages and neonatal deaths of male infants in the maternal line.

Histological criteria

Consensus definitions of histological core criteria include smallness of muscle fibres and muscle fibres with central nuclei resembling fetal myotubes. Some cases show hypotrophy of type 1 fibres. Additional criteria are a central aggregation of mitochondria in the fibres with associated highly dense oxidative enzyme staining and a corresponding lack of central staining with the ATPase reaction.

Because of its histological similarities with myotubular myopathy, congenital myotonic dystrophy has to be excluded by other than histological means (DNA analysis, electromyography in the mother). Immunohistochemical studies of desmin and vimentin may, however, contribute towards differential diagnosis. In myotonic dystrophy the involved fibres within the same fascicle appear arrested at all stages of maturation, whereas in XMTM all the fibres are morphologically relatively uniform, except for the few fibres that have a mature appearance.

Other disorders causing severe floppiness and muscle weakness, to be excluded by careful clinical and histological evaluation, are the other congenital myopathies, severe childhood spinal muscular atrophy, congenital muscular dystrophy, myasthenia and motor neuropathies. Other causes of severe hypotonia, often with normal muscle strength, include damage to the central nervous system, the Prader-Willi syndrome, connective tissue disorders and metabolic disorders.

▶ DNA Studies (NST Thomas)

Linkage analyses in XMTM families localized the gene to proximal Xq28[1–6]. Detailed studies of critical recombinant events refined this position. Physical mapping of DNA from two individuals with *de novo* interstitial deletions of Xq confirmed and refined this localization – one female with myotubular myopathy, and one male with Hunter's syndrome (iduronate sulphatase deficiency) but with no evidence of XMTM[7,8]. Physical mapping of Xq28 deletions in two unrelated males with XMTM and ambiguous external genitalia narrowed down the XMTM region still further[9]. These studies, and the possible existence of linkage heterogeneity, are summarized in the report of the 33rd ENMC international workshop[10].

This has led to the recent characterization of two candidate genes from this region, and in one of these genes a range of different mutations have been found in a number of affected males[11]. The MTM1 gene has more than 10 exons and encodes a putative tyrosine phosphatase, myotubularin. There is a highly conserved yeast homologue and three human homologues. XMTMR1 is located 100 kb telomeric of XMTM1, and the two other homologues have not yet been localized and are of unknown function[11]. Analysis of mutations in the MTM1 gene has already proved useful for unambiguous determination of carrier status in families with sporadic cases[11].

For familial cases, indirect analysis with microsatellites (the closest being DXS7423 and DXS8377) provide a useful alternative for carrier and prenatal diagnosis[12].

▶ Summary of current DNA studies

Genetic linkage analysis in several multigenerational XMTM families has identified a number of critical recombinant meioses which allow localization of the XMTM locus to the proximal Xq28 region. Physical mapping studies of DNA from an isolated case of XMTM in a girl with a *de novo* deletion of the X chromosome have confirmed this localization and defined a region of less than 2 Mb encompassing the XMTM1 gene[7]. The microsatellite marker ST71-1 has currently been shown to be the closest informative marker not showing any recombinations in previously reparted recombinant families[8].

References

1 Thomas NST, Sarfarazi M, Roberts K, *et al.* X-linked myotubular myopathy (MTM1): evidence for linkage to Xq28 DNA markers. *Cytogenet Cell Genet* 1987; 46: 704 (Abstr).

2 Darnfors C, Larsson HEB, Oldfors A, *et al.* X-linked myotubular myopathy: a linkage study. *Clin Genet* 1990; **37**: 335–40.

3 Lehesjoki A-E, Sankila E-M, Miao J, *et al.* X-linked neonatal myotubular myopathy: one recombination detected with polymorphic DNA markers from Xq28. *J Med Genet* 1990: **27**: 288–91.

4 Starr J, Lamont M, Iselius J, Harvey J, Heckmatt J. A linkage study of a large pedigree with X-linked centronuclear myopathy. *J Med Genet* 1990; **27**: 281–3.

5 Thomas NST, Williams H, Cole G, *et al.* X-linked neonatal centronuclear myotubular myopathy: evidence for linkage to Xq28 DNA marker loci. *J Med Genet* 1990; **27**: 284–7.

6 Liechti-Gallati S, Müller B, Grimm T, *et al.* X-linked centronuclear myopathy: mapping the gene to Xq28. *Neuromuscul Disord* 1991; **1**: 239–45.

7 Dahl N, Hu L-J, Chery M, *et al.* Interstitial deletion at Xq27–q28 in a girl with X-linked centronuclear myopathy. *Cytogenet Cell Genet* 1993; **64**: 181 (Abstr).

8 Dahl N, Hu L-J, Chery M, *et al.* Myotubular myopathy in a girl with a deletion at Xq27–q28 and unbalanced X-inactivation assigns the MTM1 gene to a 600 kb region. *Am J Hum Genet* 1995; **56**: 1108–15.

9 Hu L-J, Laporte J, Kress W, *et al.* Deletions in Xq28 in two boys with myotubular myopathy and abnormal genital development define a new contiguous gene syndrome in a 430 kb region. *Hum Mol Genet* 1996; **5**: 139–43.

10 Thomas NST, Wallgren-Pettersson C. Workshop report: X-linked myotubular myopathy. 33rd ENMC international workshop, Soest, The Netherlands, 9–11 June 1995. *Neuromuscul Disord* 1996; **6**: 129–32.

11 Laporte J, Hu L-J, Kretz C, *et al* A gene mutated in X-linked myotubular myopathy encodes a member of a new putative tyrosine phosphatase family conserved in yeast. *Nat Genet*, 1996; **98**: 175–82.

12 Hu L-J, Laporte J, Kioschis P, *et al.* X-linked myotubular myopathy: refinement of the gene to a 280 kb region with new and highly informative microsatellite markers. *Hum Genet*, 1996; **98**: 178–81.

This is based on reports originally published in *Neuromuscul Disord* 1994; **4(1)**: 71–74, and 1996; **6(2)**: 129–32 with permission from Pergamon Press Ltd, Headington Hill Hall, Oxford OX3 OBW, UK.

14 Nemaline Myopathy

C Wallgren-Pettersson *Dept of Medical Genetics, University of Helsinki, and the Folkhälsan Dept of Medical Genetics, Helsinki, Finland*

There are at least two forms of nemaline myopathy[1], one autosomal recessive (McKusick *256030) and one autosomal dominant (McKusick *161800). The gene for one autosomal dominant form, alpha-tropomyosin (TPM3), has been characterized, and the gene for one autosomal recessive form has been localized to chromosome 2q. No consistent qualitative differences in the clinical or histological picture have been found between the autosomal dominant and the autosomal recessive forms[2,3]. Moreover, it is unclear whether neonatally severe cases, with or without intranuclear rods, represent a separate entity.

▶ Diagnostic Criteria

Consensus core definition: Nemaline myopathy is a neuromuscular disorder characterized by muscle weakness and the presence of nemaline bodies (synonym: rods) in the muscle fibres[5,6], in the absence of other known conditions sometimes associated with rods.

▶ Clinical features

Muscle weakness

Usually most severe in the face, the neck flexors and the proximal limb muscles. In some patients there is an additional distal involvement. The extra-ocular muscles are spared. Respiratory problems are common and can be insidious. Infants commonly have feeding difficulties.

Onset

Usually in infancy, but childhood-onset as well as adult-onset cases have been described.

Inheritance

Commonly autosomal recessive, sometimes autosomal dominant. Many cases are sporadic, and the incidence of new mutations is not known.

Laboratory and neurophysiological investigations

SCK levels are normal or slightly higher (up to 5-times higher) than normal. EMG shows normal or 'myopathic' changes in young children and in proximal muscles of older patients. In distal muscles of young adult patients, EMG can show 'neuropathic' features. Nerve conduction velocities are normal.

Histological features

Light microscopy of muscle biopsy sections stained with the Gomori trichrome method shows rods in subsarcolemmal or sarcoplasmic regions of the muscle fibres. Rarely, there are intranuclear rods. There is often predominance of type 1 fibres and fibre type disproportion, or sometimes poor differentiation between fibre types. Electron microscopy shows rods with a structural periodicity resembling the lattice pattern of the Z disc. Immunohistochemical studies show the rods and the Z discs to be positive for alpha-actinin.

Exclusion criteria are sensory symptoms and signs, and other identifiable conditions sometimes associated with rod formation.

Molecular Genetic Studies

In one family, linkage of a gene (NEM1) for autosomal dominant nemaline myopathy was found to chromosome 1q, and this gene was subsequently identified as the mutated alpha-tropomyosin gene TPM3[8]. Close to 50 unrelated nemaline myopathy families have since then been tested for the presence of the TPM3 nemaline myopathy mutation but it has still only been found in the original family.

Using samples from seven European multiplex families, a recessive form of nemaline myopathy was assigned to chromosome 2q[9]. The disease gene (NEM2) was localized to a 13 cM region between the markers D2S150 and D2S141/D2S142 (internal order not determined). The maximum multipoint lod score, 5.34, was found for a point corresponding to the marker D2S151.

References

1 Dubowitz V. *Muscle disorders in childhood*, 2nd ed, WB Saunders: London, 1995, 147–52.

2 Wallgren-Pettersson C. Congenital nemaline myopathy: A clinical follow-up study of twelve patients. *J Neurol Sci* 1989; **89**: 1–14.

3 Wallgren-Pettersson C, Kääriäinen H, Rapola J, *et al.* Genetics of congenital nemaline myopathy – a study of ten families. *J Med Genet* 1990; **27**: 480–7.

4 Barohn R, Jackson CE, Kagan-Hallet KS. Neonatal nemaline myopathy with abundant intranuclear rods. *Neuromuscul Disord* 1994; **4**: 513–20.

5 Conen PE, Murphy EG, Donohue WL. Light and electron microscopic studies of "myogranules" in a child with hypotonia and muscle weakness. *Can Med Assoc J* 1963; **89**: 983–6.

6 Shy GM, Engel WK, Somers JE, *et al.* Nemaline myopathy. A new congenital myopathy. *Brain* 1963; **86**: 793–810.

7 Laing NG, Majda BT, Akkari PA, *et al.* Assignment of a gene (NEM1) for autosomal dominant nemaline myopathy to chromosome 1. *Am J Hum Genet* 1992; **50**: 576–83.

8 Laing NG, Wilton SD, Akkari PA, *et al.* A mutation in the alpha-tropomyosin gene TPM3 associated with autosomal dominant nemaline myopathy NEM1. *Nat Genet* 1995; **9**: 75–9.

9 Wallgren-Pettersson C, Avela K, Marchand S, *et al.* A gene for autosomal recessive nemaline myopathy assigned to chromosome 2q by linkage analysis. *Neuromuscul Disord* 1995; 6: 441–3.

This is based on the report of the 40th ENMC International Workshop: Nemaline myopathy shortly to be published in *Neuromuscul Disord* with permission from Pergamon Press Ltd, Headington Hill Hall, Oxford OX3 OBW, UK.

15 Mini Core Disease and Central Core Disease

LT Middleton *The Cyprus Institute of Neurology and Genetics, Nicosia, Cyprus*

H Moser *Universitäts Kinderklinik, Inselspital, Bern, Switzerland*

▶ Diagnostic Criteria

Here are presented the diagnostic criteria for two rare neuromuscular disorders: mini core disease and central core disease.

Mini core disease

1 Inheritance: autosomal recessive; isolated; (autosomal dominant?).
2 Age at onset: infancy; rarely 2–12 years of age.
3 Primary clinical criteria:
Generalized muscle weakness and hypotonia, proximal muscles more involved than distal.
4 Additional features:
  a Ptosis, facial and extra-ocular muscle weakness.
  b Distal involvement, joint contractures.
  c Cardiac abnormalities.
5 Evolution: non-progressive.
6 Histology:
  a Mini cores demonstrated by oxidative enzyme reaction, usually measure 7 μ in width and up to 75 μ in length. Usually multiple and found in both type 1 and type 2 fibres
  b Distinctive electronmicroscopy
  c Type 1 predominance.
7 Other laboratory investigations:
  a SCK normal or mildly elevated (three-times normal)
  b EMG normal or myopathic.
8 Exclusion criteria:
  a CNS dysfunction.
  b Vision/hearing defects.
9 Note: adult cardiomyopathy with mini cores?

Central core disease

1 Inheritance: autosomal dominant; isolated; (autosomal recessive?).
2 Age at onset: infancy or, rarely, adult life.
3 Primary clinical criteria:
   a Hypotonia, delayed motor milestones.
   b Generalized muscle weakness, proximal muscles more involved than distal.
   c Legs more involved than arms.
   d Normal intelligence.
4 Additional features:
   a Facial, sternomastoid and trapezius muscles may be involved but not extra-ocular muscles.
   b Skeletal abnormalities – flat feet, pes cavus, kyphoscoliosis, congenital hip dislocation.
   c Susceptibility to malignant hyperthermia.
5 Evolution: non-progressive, can be slowly progressive.
6 Histology:
   a Central, well demarcated cores visible with oxidative enzyme reactions and confined to type 1 fibres. The cores are long and may be eccentric or multiple.
   b Distinctive electronmicroscopy.
   c Type 1 fibre predominance.
   d Minor myopathic features may occur but necrosis or regeneration is rare.
7 Other laboratory investigations:
   a SCK is normal or slightly increased (less than three-times normal).
   b EMG is normal or myopathic.

This is based on a report originally published in *Neuromuscul Disord* 1995; **4(3)**: 273–5 with permission from Pergamon Press Ltd, Headington Hill Hall, Oxford OX3 OBW, UK.

16 Desminopathies

HH Goebel *Division of Neuropathology, University Medical Centre, Mainz, Germany*

M Fardeau *INSERM, 'Développement, Pathologie, Régéneration du Système Neuromusculaire', Paris, France*

Introduction

Desmin, the intermediate filament of skeletal (and cardiac) muscle fibres abnormally accumulates in certain myopathies – sometimes associated with cardiomyopathy – sporadically or in a familial fashion. These are called desminopathies or desmin 'storage' myopathies.

Three groups of neuromuscular conditions fall into this category:

a The autosomal dominant form with accumulation of granulo-filamentous material (with or without evidence of neuropathic involvement)[1–11].
b The autosomal-dominant form with cytoplasmic/spheroid inclusion bodies[12–24].
c The autosomal-recessive form with 'Mallory body'-like inclusion bodies or hyaline/desmin plaques[25–27].

The separation and final definition of these neuromuscular disorders as nosological entities will be complete upon their gene identification. Their current separation into three categories is based on morphological features.

Exclusion Criteria

Excluded are those neuromuscular conditions where desmin occurs as evidence of regeneration or immaturity in certain congenital myopathies, e.g. myotubular and nemaline myopathies.

Diagnostic Criteria

Autosomal dominant form with accumulation of granulo-filamentous material (with or without evidence of neuropathic involvement)[1–11]

Age of onset
Most often early to middle adulthood.

Inheritance
Autosomal dominant.

Clinical symptoms

Chest pain and distal muscle weakness and atrophy[4], gait abnormalities[10], cardiac insufficency[11], velopharyngeal muscles involved[4]. Normal eye movements.

Progression

Slowly progressive, but marked by cardiac death.

Cardiac involvement

Constant: hypertrophic cardiomyopathy and/or cardiac arrhythmias.

Electromyography

Myopathic or mixed pattern.

SCK

Normal or mildly elevated.

Additional signs

Lens opacities[4], neuropathy[2,10], intestinal malabsorption and pseudo-obstruction[1].

Morphology

Diffuse accumulation of granulofilamentous material, the filaments containing desmin distributed in a garland-like fashion, subsarcolemmally and among myofibrils with little or no disruption of sarcomeres[4], desmin being abnormally phosphorylated[2,9]. In addition, dystrophin[6,8] and vimentin[6] may be associated. Moreover, cytoplasmic bodies may also be present[2,3,5]. Increase of desmin intermediate filaments is also encountered in cardiac myocytes[1] or granulo-filamentous material in cardiomyocytes[2]. Affected nerves show giant axons owing to the accumulation of neurofilaments[2,10].

▶ Autosomal-dominant form with cytoplasmic/spheroid inclusion bodies[12–24]

Age of onset

Usually adolescence or adulthood, occasionally childhood[21].

Inheritance

Autosomal dominant, sporadic, (autosomal-recessive?).

Clinical symptoms

Muscle weakness, in some families distal, in others generalized or proximal, respiratory insufficiency[15], no involvement of eye muscles.

Progression

Slowly, but occasionally accelerated by respiratory insufficiency.

Cardiac involvement

Occasionally[18].

Electromyography
Myopathic.

SCK
Normal or mildly elevated.

Additional signs
Fatigability after exertion, dysphonia, and dysphagia[24].

Morphology
Muscle fibres of index patients and other family members show desmin-related inclusions, cytoplasmic bodies[15], spheroid bodies[16,19], spheroid-cytoplasmic complexes, or sarcoplasmic bodies[18]. Cytoplasmic bodies are well circumscribed and consist of a core of dense granular material surrounded by a halo of intermediate (desmin-positive) filaments. The spheroid bodies are larger and display a more mixed pattern of granular material and filaments[19], but the terms cytoplasmic and spheroid have been used interchangeably[15]. Large masses of these inclusions are referred to as spheroid–cytoplasmic complexes. In the modified trichrome preparation these inclusion bodies are sometimes red, sometimes greenish. Additional proteins include dystrophin[12], actin, and utrophin[14]. In some instances desmin could not be verified in cytoplasmic bodies[20,24].

Autosomal-recessive form with 'Mallory body'-like inclusion bodies or hyaline/desmin plaques[25–27]

Age of onset
Early childhood.

Inheritance
Autosomal-recessive

Clinical findings
Proximal or generalized weakness including respiratory failure, facial weakness, but no eye muscle involvement, high-arched palate, scoliosis, lordosis, no cardiac involvement.

Progression
Sometimes slowly, but often rapidly to death.

Electromyogram
Myopathic.

SCK
Mildly elevated.

Morphology
Desmin-positive inclusions with granular material, intermediate filaments, and helical filaments called 'Mallory body'-like inclusion bodies or hyaline plaques.

References

1 Ariza A, Coll J, Fernández-Figueras MT, *et al.* Desmin myopathy: a multisystem disorder involving skeletal, cardiac, and smooth muscle. *Hum Pathol* 1995; **26**: 1032–7.

2 Bertini E, Bosman C, Ricci E, *et al.* Neuromyopathy and restrictive cardiomyopathy with accumulation of intermediate filaments: a clinical, morpholigical and biochemical study. *Acta Neuropathol (Berl)* 1991; **81**: 632–40.

3 Cameron CHS, Mirakhur M, Allen IV. Desmin myopathy with cardiomyopathy. *Acta Neuropathol (Berl)* 1995; **89**: 560–6.

4 Fardeau M, Godet-Guillain J, Tomé FMS, *et al.* Une nouvelle affection musculaire familiale, définie par l'accumulation intrasarco-plasmique d'un matériel granulo-filamentaire dense en microscopie électronique. *Rev Neurol (Paris)* 1978; **134**: 411–25.

5 Goebel HH, Voit T, Warlo I, *et al.* Immunohistologic and electron microscopic abnormalities of desmin and dystrophin in familial cardiomyopathy and myopathy. *Rev Neurol (Paris)* 1994; **150**: 452–9.

6 Helliwell TR, Green ART, Green A, *et al.* Hereditary distal myopathy with granulo-filamentous cytoplasmic inclusions containing desmin, dystrophin and vimentin. *J Neurol Sci* 1994; **124**: 174–87.

7 Horowitz SH, Schmalbruch H. Autosomal dominant distal myopathy with desmin storage: a clinicopathologic and electrophysiologic study of a large kinship. *Muscle Nerve* 1994; **17**: 151–60.

8 Prelle A, Moggio M, Comi GP, *et al.* Congenital myopathy associated with abnormal accumulation of desmin and dystrophin. *Neuromuscul Disord* 1992; **2**: 169–75.

9 Rappaport L, Contard F, Samuel JL, *et al.* Storage of phosphorylated desmin in a familial myopathy. *FEBS Lett* 1988; **231**: 421–5.

10 Sabatelli M, Bertini E, Ricci E, *et al.* Peripheral neuropathy with giant axons and cardiomyopathy associated with desmin type intermediate filaments in skeletal muscle. *J Neurol Sci* 1992; **109**: 1–10.

11 Vajsar J, Becker LE, Freedom RM, *et al.* Familial desminopathy: myopathy with accumulation of desmin-type intermediate filaments. *J Neurol Neurosurg Psychiatry* 1993; **56**: 644–8.

12 Caron A, Chapon F, Berthelin CH, *et al.* Inclusions in familial cytoplasmic body myopathy are stained by anti-dystrophin antibodies. *Neuromuscul Disord* 1993; **3**: 541–6.

13 Caron A, Viader F, Lechevalier B, *et al.* Cytoplasmic body myopathy: familial cases with accumulation of desmin and dystrophin. An immunohistochemical, immunoelectron microscopic and biochemical study. *Acta Neuropathol (Berl)* 1995; **90**: 150–7.

14 Caron A, Lechevalier B, Chapon F. Immunohistochemical, immunoelectron microscopic and biochemical study of a familial cytoplasmic body myopathy. *Neuropathol Appl Neurobiol* 1996; **22 (Suppl 1)**: 110 (P168).

15 Chapon F, Viader F, Fardeau M, *et al.* Myopathie familiale avec inclusions de type <<corps cytoplasmique>> (ou <<sphéroides>>) révélée par une insuffisance respiratoire. *Rev Neurol (Paris)* 1989; **145**: 460–5.

16 Clark JR, D'Agostino AN, Wilson J, *et al.* Autosomal dominant myofibrillar inclusion body myopathy: clinical, histologic, histochemical, and ultrastructural characteristics. *Neurology* 1978; **28**: 399.

17 Dickoff DJ. Adult onset of inherited myopathies. *Prog Clin Neurosci* 1988; **1**: 65–80.
18 Edström L, Thornell LE, Eriksson A. A new type of hereditary distal myopathy with characteristic sarcoplasmic bodies and intermediate (skeletin) filaments. *J Neurol Sci* 1980; **47**: 171–90.
19 Goebel HH, Muller J, Gillen HW, *et al.* Autosomal dominant "spheroid body myopathy". *Muscle Nerve* 1978; **1**: 14–26.
20 Guimaraes A, Rebelo O, Magalhaes M. Familial cytoplasmic body myopathy. *Neuropathol Appl Neurobiol* 1996; **22 (Suppl 1)**: 4 (C12).
21 Mizuno Y, Nakamura Y, Komiya K. The spectrum of cytoplasmic body myopathy: report of a congenital severe case. *Brain Dev* 1989; **11**: 20–25.
22 Navarro C, Teijeira S, Fernández JM, *et al.* Desmin myopathy. Report on two cases with different clinical phenotype and review of the literature. *Clin Neuropathol* 1994; **13**: 105.
23 Pellissier JF, Pouget J, Charpin C, *et al.* Myopathy associated with desmin type intermediate filaments. *J Neurol Sci* 1989; **89**: 49–61.
24 Pellisier JF, Baeta AM, Cassote E, *et al.* Familial desmin myopathies. *Neuropathol Appl Neurobiol* 1996; **22 (Suppl 1)**: 109 (P164).
25 Fidzianska A, Goebel HH, Osborn M, *et al.* Mallory body-like inclusions in a hereditary congenital neuromuscular disease. *Muscle Nerve* 1983; **6**: 195–200.
26 Fidzianska A, Ryniewicz B, Barcikowska M, *et al.* A new familial congenital myopathy in children with desmin and dystrophin reacting plaques. *J Neurol Sci* 1995; **131**: 88–95.
27 Goebel HH, Lenard HG, Langenbeck U, *et al.* A form of congenital muscular dystrophy. *Brain Dev* 1980; **2**: 387–400.

This is based on a report originally published in *Neuromuscul Disord* 1995; **5(2)**: 161–6 and on the report of the 36th ENMC International Workshop: Familial desmin-related myopathies and cardiomyopathies shortly to be published with permission from Pergamon Press Ltd, Headington Hill Hall, Oxford OX3 0BW, UK.

17 Inclusion Body Myositis

JJ Vershuuren, UA Badrising, AR Wintzen *Dept of Neurology, Leiden University Hospital, Leiden, The Netherlands*
BGM van Engelen *Dept of Neurology, University Hospital Nijmegen, Nijmegen, The Netherlands*
H van der Hoeven *Dept of Neurology, University Hospital Groningen, Groningen, The Netherlands*
J Hoogendijk *Dept of Neurology, University Hospital Utrecht, Utrecht, The Netherlands*

▶ Diagnostic Criteria

Here are presented the diagnostic criteria for inclusion body myositis (IBM). These criteria are the result of a consensus Workshop organized by the Dutch Neuromuscular Research Support Centre in April 1996.

Criteria are defined as a combination of elements. Depending on the combination of elements which are fulfilled, the diagnosis of IBM can be definite, probable or possible.

None of the clinical or laboratory elements are by themselves pathognomonic for IBM. According to diagnostic criteria for IBM, published in 1995, a definite diagnosis of IBM depends completely on muscle biopsy features. None of the clinical or laboratory features were mandatory if the muscle biopsy was diagnostic[1]. Recent reports, however, stress that IBM might have a characteristic pattern of muscle weakness, involving the quadriceps femoris muscles in the lower limbs and the forearm muscles, particularly the finger flexors, in the upper limbs[2,3,4]. Therefore, it was decided that clinical features should have a more prominent role in the diagnostic criteria. The following diagnostic criteria include the possibility to make a diagnosis of definite IBM based on the typical pattern of weakness in combination with a muscle biopsy which shows inflammation and vacuolated fibres, but in which the presence of tubulofilaments or amyloid has not been demonstrated.

Elements

1 Muscular weakness is present[1,5,6].
Comment. Weakness can be present in proximal, as well as in distal limb muscles. Weakness usually starts in the lower limbs, involving particularly the quadriceps muscle. Occasionally dysphagia is the first symptom. Weakness is often asymmetrical. Facial muscles are involved in the disease process, but external eye muscles are spared. Myalgia is unusual, but can incidentally be present.

2 Weakness of the forearm muscles, particularly the finger flexor, and/or wrist flexor muscles more than the wrist extensor muscles, is typical in the disease. This has been reported as one of the first symptoms, even before the disease process results in a more generalized weakness[2,3,4].
Comment. The predominant involvement of these muscles is remarkable as compared to other muscle diseases, and can be a valuable diagnostic clue. Some recent studies report weakness in these muscles in about 80% of patients.

3 The disease has a slowly progressive course, during which the weakness extends to other muscles, including the facial muscles[4,6].
Comment. The presence of signs and/or symptoms 5 years or more before a diagnosis of IBM is made is not exceptional: a range of 0.5 to 30 years has been reported in the literature[7]. Spontaneous stabilization of the disease has never been documented, but this possibility has not been excluded. Decreased or absent tendon reflexes can be found in weak muscles.

4 IBM is most often a disease of middle-aged or elderly men[4,5].
Comment. About 80% of the patients are 50 years or older at the time of diagnosis. IBM can be found 2–4 times more often in males than females.

5 IBM is a sporadic disease[1,5].
Comment. One report described an unusual type of IBM in two sisters. The muscle biopsies showed infiltrates, which are not found in familial inclusion body myopathy. The myositis improved during therapy with prednisolone and was described as 'glucocorticoid-sensitive hereditary inclusion body myositis'[8].

6 SCK is normal or mildly to moderately increased[4,5].
Comment. SCK is most often 2–5-times normal, and in a minority of patients up to 12-times increased. In some atypical cases higher values have been reported[9]. In 10–20% of patients normal SCK activity is found.

7 Electromyography is 'myopathic' or 'mixed neuromyopathic'. In a minority of patients electromyographic studies only have 'neuropathic' features.
Comment. Fibrillation potentials and/or positive sharp waves can be recorded in most patients. In most patients motor unit potentials are 'myopathic' (small/short), but 'neuropathic' (large/long) potentials can occur. A mild decrease of nerve conduction velocity does not exclude a diagnosis of IBM.

8 A muscle biopsy shows mononuclear inflammatory cellular infiltrates, located predominantly or exclusively in the endomysium, and invasion of non-necrotic muscle fibres by mononuclear cells[10,11].
Comment. Necrotic muscle fibres can be present; atrophic, often angular, muscle fibres are common; eosinophilic inclusions in the sarcoplasma may be found. There is controversy if muscle fibres from patients with IBM do express HLA-type 1 molecules[12,13].

9 Some non-necrotic muscle fibres contain rimmed vacuoles (at least 1 per 1000 muscle fibres)[5,14].
Comment. Vacuoles often contain, or are rimmed by, basophilic material. Some authors describe amyloid in non-necrotic vacuolated muscle fibres, using a fluorescent Congo-red staining method.

10 Vacuolated muscle fibres contain cytoplasmic tubulofilaments, with diameters of about 16–21 nm. Similar tubulofilaments are also found in the nucleus[1].

11 In muscle biopsies of IBM patients ragged red fibres can be found[1,15].
Comment. Paracrystalline structures can be found in muscle mitochondria.

12 Immunosuppressive treatment does not result in stabilization or remission of the disease process[4,5,6,16,17].

Comment. Some reports indicate that patients may benefit from prolonged treatment[9,18].

13 Inclusion body myositis occurs in association with other, especially autoimmune, diseases such as systemic lupus erythematodes, mixed connective tissue disease, scleroderma, idiopathic thrombocytopenic purpura, thyroid dysfunction, sarcoidosis[5,19].

Assessment

The diagnosis is **definite** when:

a 1, 2, 3, 5, 8, 9 or 1, 3, 5, 8, 9, 10 are fulfilled.
b 12 confirms the diagnosis.
c 4, 6, 11, and 13 are compatible with the diagnosis.

The diagnosis is **probable** when:

a 1, 2, 3, 5, 8 or 1, 3, 5, 8, 9 are fulfilled.
b 4, 6, 11, 12, 13 are compatible with the diagnosis.

The diagnosis is **possible** when:

a 1, 3, 4, 8, 12 are fulfilled.
b 4, 6, 13 are compatible with the diagnosis.

References

1 Griggs RC, Askanas V, DiMauro S, *et al.* Inclusion body myositis and myopathies. *Ann Neurol* 1995; **38**: 705–13.

2 Sekul E, Chow C, Dalakas MC. Magnetic resonance imaging (MRI) of the forearm as a diagnostic aid in patients with inclusion body myositis (IBM). *Neurology* 1994; **44**: A310.

3 Amato AA, Gronseth GS, Jackson CE, *et al.* Inclusion-body myositis: pattern of weakness and clinical features and evidence supporting the diagnosis of probable inclusion-body myositis. *Neurology* 1996; **46**: A486.

4 Lindberg C, Persson LI, Bjorklander J, *et al.* Inclusion body myositis: clinical, morphological, physiological and laboratory findings in 18 cases. *Acta Neurol Scand* 1994; **89**: 123–31.

5 Lotz BP, Engel AG, Nishino H, *et al.* Inclusion body myositis. Observations in 40 patients. *Brain* 1989; **112**: 727–47.

6 Beyenburg S, Zierz S, Jerusalem F. Inclusion body myositis: clinical and histopathological features of 36 patients. *Clin Invest* 1993; **71**: 351–61.

7 Riggs JE, Schocher SS, Gutmann L, *et al.* Childhood inclusion body myositis mimicking limb-girdle muscular dystrophy. *J Child Neurol* 1989; **4**: 283–5.

8 Naumann M, Reichmann H, Goebel HH, *et al.* Glucocorticoid-sensitive hereditary inclusion body myositis. *J Neurol* 1996; **243**: 126–30.

9 Jongen PJ, ter Laak HJ, van der Putte LB. Inclusion body myositis responding to long-term chlorambucil treatment. *J Rheumatol* 1995; **22**: 576–8.

10 Engel AG, Arahata K. Monoclonal antibody analysis of mononuclear cells in myopathies. II: phenotypes of autoinvasive cells in polymyositis and inclusion body myositis. *Ann Neurol* 1984; **16**: 209–15.

11 Ned Pruit IIJ, Showalter CJ, Engel AG. Sporadic inclusion body myositis: counts of different types of abnormal fibres. *Ann Neurol* 1996; **39**: 139–43.

12 McDouall RM, Dunn MJ, Dubowitz V. Expression of class I and class II MHC antigens in neuromuscular diseases. *J Neurol Sci* 1989; **89**: 213–26.

13 Karpati G, Pouliot G, Carpenter S. Expression of immunoreactive major histocompatibility complex products in human skeletal muscles. *Ann Neurol* 1988; **23**: 64–72.

14 Jongen PJ, ter Laak HJ, Stadhouders AM. Rimmed basophilic vacuoles and filamentous inclusions in neuromuscular disorders. *Neuromuscul Disord* 1995; **5**: 31–8.

15 Rifai Z, Welle S, Kamp C, *et al.* Ragged red fibres in normal ageing and inflammatory myopathy. *Ann Neurol* 1995; **37**: 24–29.

16 Amato AA, Barohn RJ, Jackson CE, *et al.* Inclusion body myositis: treatment with intravenous immunogobulin. *Neurol* 1994; **44**: 1516–8.

17 Dalakas MC, Dambrosia JM, Sekul EA, *et al.* The efficacy of high dose intravenous immunoglobulin (IvIg) in patients with inclusion body myositis (IBM). *Neurol* 1994; **45 (Suppl 4)**: A208.

18 Sayers ME, Chou SM, Calabrese LH. Inclusion body myositis: Analysis of 32 cases. *J Rheumatol* 1992; **19**: 1385–9.

18 Mitochondrial Myopathies

L Bindoff *Dept of Neurology, Middlesborough General Hospital, Middlesborough, UK*
G Brown *Dept of Biochemistry, University of Oxford, Oxford, UK*
J Poulton *Dept of Paediatrics, John Radcliffe Hospital, Oxford, UK*

▶ Introduction

It is important to recognize that mitochondrial diseases are systemic conditions and not confined to the neuromuscular system (NMS). Many of them manifest as disease of the NMS however, and these will be discussed here. Attempts at classifying mitochondrial myopathies (MM) have used clinical, biochemical and more recently genetic criteria, but no one category alone is sufficient, and a combination of two or more is required. Certain phenotypes are almost always associated with mitochondrial dysfunction, whilst in others mitochondrial dysfunction is one of several potential causes. The combination of clinical phenotype and either biochemical or genetic evidence of significant mitochondrial dysfunction is sufficient to diagnose MM[1], but the important qualification is the degree of the abnormalities. Identifying mitochondrial dysfunction as the primary cause must take into account that minor biochemical abnormalities have been detected in a variety of conditions (ageing, Huntington's chorea, Parkinson's disease) and mutated mitochondrial DNA (mtDNA) can be found in supposedly normal but aged individuals. In order to provide some guidelines we have suggested levels of abnormality considered significant. However, this may exclude some patients with obvious MM based on widely accepted criteria, a clear reflection that the classification remains imprecise. Diagnostic criteria are given for syndromes recognized as mitochondrial disorders, and laboratory and genetic criteria.

▶ Clinical Criteria

Several clinical syndromes have been defined which are almost always due to mitochondrial dysfunction[1]. Although many patients fit clearly into one or other of these syndromes, considerable overlap can occur between them.

▶ Kearns–Sayre syndrome (KSS)

I The cardinal features are progressive external ophthalmoplegia (PEO), retinal pigmentary degeneration and an onset before 15 years of age.
C Additional features may include heart block, elevated CSF protein, ataxia,

myopathy, dementia, small stature, sensory neural deafness and diabetes mellitus. Rarely other endocrine dysfunction is found.

I Muscle biopsy will almost always show cytochrome oxidase (COX) negative fibres and ragged red fibres (RRF) in adults but RRFs are uncommon in young children.

I Genetic analysis demonstrates rearrangement of mtDNA including a tandem duplication[2] and/or deletion[3]. Whilst the majority are sporadic, family history may rarely be positive for maternal transmission.

Chronic progressive external ophthalmoplegia (CPEO)

C This is a more loosely defined syndrome, but may contain many of the features described for Kearns–Sayre syndrome with a later onset.

I Most patients have a mild proximal myopathy in addition to ophthalmoplegia, and might have pigmentary retinopathy, ataxia, sensory neural deafness, mild pyramidal or extrapyramidal features.

I Onset is later than Kearns–Sayre syndrome and may be as late as the fifth or sixth decade.

I Muscle-biopsy shows COX negative fibres and RRF and mtDNA analysis will show a single large scale rearrangement in approximately 50% (sporadic cases).

I Autosomal dominant inheritance with evidence of multiple deletions on Southern blotting and PCR analysis of muscle is characteristic of ADPEO (autosomal dominant progressive external ophthalmoplegia)[4]. Although documented in a small proportion of patients with CPEO it is probably under-diagnosed.

I In a significant proportion of the other patients, point mutations of mtDNA can be defined, the most common being position 3243 (see below) and maternal relatives may be affected.

Mitochondrial encephalomyopathy, lactic acidosis and stroke-like episodes (MELAS)

I The defining feature of this syndrome is recurrent stroke-like episodes. The lesions are not related to vascular territories and often involve the parieto-occipital regions, presenting with visual abnormalities.

I Myopathy, lactic acidosis (predominantly found in CSF) and encephalopathy are the other parts of the syndrome, but recent evidence demonstrates the inconsistency with which all four features are found together.

C In its pure form, MELAS often affects young children and seizures are the commonest presenting features. Patients are usually small, may have dementia, sensory neural deafness and a family history with maternal inheritance.

I Muscle biopsy is abnormal in the majority showing both COX positive and negative RRF and sometimes strongly succinate dehydrogenase positive vessels (SSVs). The majority of cases are caused by a point mutation in mtDNA at position 3243[5] although other mutations have also been described such as 3271, 8344, 3260[6] and large scale re-arrangements.

Myoclonus, epilepsy with ragged red fibres (MERRF)

I The combination of myclonus, epilepsy and RRF myopathy are the cardinal signs, but common additional features are deafness, ataxia and dementia.

C Less commonly, small stature and lipomatosis can be found.

I As suggested by the defining features RRF and COX negative fibres are identifiable in muscle, and genetic analysis demonstrates that a large percentage of the cases can be defined by a point mutation at position 8344[7]. A second point mutation at 8356 has also been identified[8].

Pure myopathy

This can be divided into infantile and child/adult forms.

Infantile pure myopathy

Two forms of this rare condition are recognized – lethal and benign.

I Both types may be accompanied by renal tubulopathies and/or hepatic dysfunction.

C Most cases of mtDNA depletion fall into the fatal group.

Benign infantile myopathy (BIM)

I This presents at birth with hypotonia, breathing and feeding difficulties plus profound lactic acidosis. This condition spontaneously improves, usually from around 6 to 9 months although it can be later.

C If these children can be supported appropriately then they will survive.

I The condition is usually associated with a deficiency of cytochrome c oxidase[9] perhaps due to a fetal isoform. Muscle from these infants shows a uniform loss of COX activity but not the mosaic seen in other MM. Improvement coincides with normalization of COX activity.

C Inheritance is probably autosomal recessive, but detailed genetic information is lacking. Some cases of mtDNA depletion may be included in this group.

Lethal infantile myopathy (LIM)

I Often presents soon after birth, usually within 2 to 3 weeks, with severe lactic acidosis associated with hypotonia, respiratory and feeding difficulties.

C These infants usually die within months and Fanconi syndrome may be prominent.

I Muscle biopsy once again shows a uniform loss of COX activity[9], but in this group other biochemical defects e.g. loss of complex I or complex III activity, have also been described.

C Most cases of mtDNA depletion fall into this fatal group and inheritance is probably autosomal recessive in most cases[10].

Child/adult pure myopathy[1]

I This is a progressive, usually painless myopathy which can mimic other muscle diseases such as limb-girdle or fascioscapular humeral dystrophies. Fatigue may be prominent, serum lactate is often mildly elevated and muscle biopsy shows RRF, frequently with a mosaic of COX positive and negative fibres.

C No pattern of inheritance is common and a variety of mtDNA defects have been described, usually as single cases or single families.

Other syndromes

Apart from the well defined syndromes, there are several descriptions of encephalomyopathies and cardiomyopathies due to primary mitochondrial disease which have been investigated in detail.

Encephalopathies

I The major manifestations are seizures, encephalopathy, dementia or development regression and ataxia.

I The presence of muscle involvement provides a convenient avenue for diagnosis and the finding of significant numbers of COX negative fibres (see later) provides the diagnosis.

I Genetic analysis has shown a number of point mutations in mtDNA.

Leigh's encephalopathy

I Leigh's encephalopathy is a pathological diagnosis based on characteristic cystic cavitation with vascular proliferation, neuronal loss and demyelination in the midbrain and basal ganglia[11]. Patients present with lactic acidosis, progressive psychomotor retardation and brain stem and/or basal ganglia dysfunction.

I Severe muscle specific COX deficiency with autosomal recessive inheritance or pyruvate dehydrogenase deficiency with X-linked inheritance are common findings. Other patients may have high levels of one of a number of point mutations in mtDNA (most commonly at bp 8993).

Cardiomyopathies

I In cardiomyopathies with a myopathic component the histochemical and genetic findings are similar to the encephalopathies.

Neurogenic weakness ataxia and retinitis pigmentosa (NARP)

I Weakness is due to an axonal sensorimotor neuropathy and muscle biopsy is frequently normal (histology and biochemical findings).

I Retinitis pigmentosa, mental retardation/developmental delay, ataxia and raised lactate are common features.

I This syndrome is associated with a mtDNA point mutation at position 8993[11,12]. Manifestations are very variable. This disease is commonly identified in families with one or more members presenting as maternally inherited Leigh's syndrome (MILS).

Laboratory Criteria

Morphological and general biochemical indicators

I The single most important investigation is muscle biopsy with good histochemical analysis. In the vast majority of adult cases with the conditions described above, there will be subsarcolemmal accumulation of mitochondria (RRF) and/or fibres which lack cytochrome c oxidase (COX negative fibres). This is less consistent in the paediatric age range.

E Studies in aged muscle suggest that apparently normal individuals may have 1–2% COX negative fibres, but usually show no evidence whatsoever of RRF. Both have been found in inflammatory conditions, but these should be distinguishable on clinical grounds. Thus, we feel the presence of COX negative/

RRF at levels higher than 2% in the appropriate clinical setting is evidence of mitochondrial myopathy.

C COX negative fibres can occur without RRF. This can be the case in all the conditions noted above, but is certainly the case in Leigh's disease due to systemic COX deficiency and in some pure myopathies which may present with isolated loss of COX activity which is uniformly distributed in all muscle cells.

C The presence of a raised SCK, EMG evidence of myopathy and raised lactate (in serum or CSF) are all important indicators but insufficient alone to be diagnostic of MM. In patients with renal tubulopathies, urinary lactate may be raised despite a normal blood lactate. All of these parameters may be normal and this may provide the major clue to the presence of a metabolic myopathy in a patient with muscle symptoms.

Specific biochemical criteria

C *In vitro* assays of respiratory chain function are technically difficult and not universally available. Techniques vary between centres, making comparisons difficult (particularly in the case of complex I activity). Polarographic studies have certain advantages but require fresh tissue in relatively large amount.

I Myopathies in which morphological changes (RRF or COX negative fibres) are associated with reduced activities of electron transport chain components can still be defined as primarily mitochondrial. Because of the variation in absolute activities, it may be more helpful to express results as ratios between the different complexes and/or between the complexes and a mitochondrial marker enzyme such as citrate synthase. The level of deficiency of respiratory chain complex activity should be clearly below the control range in the appropriate tissue, i.e. often below 20% for at least one of the complexes or ratios measured.

C The expression of respiratory chain defects in cultured cells may be unstable. Normal respiratory enzyme activities do not preclude mitochondrial dysfunction even when the tissue tested expresses the disease.

Genetic Criteria

Rearrangement of mtDNA

I The presence of deletion[3], duplication or a mixture of these species in addition to wild type[2] is regarded as pathological and is almost always seen in patients with KSS.

E Deletions of mtDNA (particularly the so called 'common deletion') are pathological in the appropriate clinical setting e.g. KSS, CPEO, but have been found in low levels (< 1%) in ageing tissue, particularly post mitotic tissue such as skeletal muscle, but also in low levels in oocytes. Levels that are undetectable by Southern blotting are generally considered not to be pathological.

Point mutations of mtDNA

I A variety of pathological mutations have been identified, some of which have been verified as causative by rho zero cell experiments (the best established are: 3243, 3252, 3260, 3271, 8344, 8356). The level of these mutations may vary between affected individuals and between tissues in an affected individual but their presence, in the appropriate clinical setting, is diagnostic of mitochondrial disease. Currently, these mutations should be viewed as potentially pathological and transmissable in females even if present in apparently normal individuals at levels > 1%.

I There are now more than 30 mtDNA point mutations described in the literature, many in single cases or in single families. It is impossible to give classification for all without verification (e.g. rho zero experiments or correlation of level of mutant with the phenotype of single cells) but it is likely that most, if not all, are pathological.

References

1 Jackson M, Schaefer J, Johnson M, *et al.* Presentation and clinical investigation of mitochondrial respiratory chain disease: a study of 52 patients. *Brain* 1995; **118**: 339–57.

2 Poulton J, Deadman NE, Bindoff L, *et al.* Families of mtDNA re-arrangements can be detected in patients with mtDNA deletions: duplications may be a transient intermediate form. *Hum Mol Genet* 1993; **2(1)**: 23–30.

3 Holt IJ, Harding AE, Morgan-Hughes JA. Deletions in muscle mitochondrial DNA in patients with mitochondrial myopathies. *Nature* 1988; **331**: 717–9.

4 Zeviani M, Servidei S, Gellera C, *et al.* An autosomal dominant disorder with multiple deletions of mitochondrial DNA starting at the D-loop region. *Nature* 1989; **339**: 309–11.

5 Goto YI, Nonaka I, Horai S. A mutation in the tRNA leu(UUR) gene associated with the MELAS subgroup of mitochondrial encephalomyopathies. *Nature* 1990; **348**: 651–3.

6 Zeviani M, Gellera C, Antozzi C, *et al.* Maternally inherited myopathy and cardiomyopathy: association with mutation in mitochondrial DNA tRNA (Leu)(UUR). *Lancet* 1991; **338**: 143–7.

7 Shoffner JM, Lott MT, Lezza AM, *et al.* Myoclonic epilepsy and ragged-red fiber disease (MERRF) is associated with a mitochondrial DNA tRNA(Lys) mutation. *Cell* 1990; **61**: 931–7.

8 Zeviani M, Muntoni F, Saravese N, *et al.* A MERRF/MELAS overlap syndrome associated with a new point mutation in the mitochondrial DNA $tRNA^{lys}$ gene. *Eur J Hum Genet* 1993; **1**: 80–87.

9 Bresolin N, Gonano F, Comi G. Cytochrome-c oxidase deficiencies. In: Darley-Usmar V, Schapira A, Eds. *Mitochondria: DNA, proteins and disease.* London: Portland Press 1994.

10 Moraes CT, Shanske S, Tritschler HG, *et al.* mtDNA depletion with variable tissue expression: a novel genetic abnormality in mitochondrial disease. *Am J Hum Genet* 1991; **48**: 492–501.

11 Rahman S, Blok R, Dahl H, *et al.* Leigh syndrome: clinical features and biochemical and DNA abnormalities. *Ann Neurol* 1996; **39**: 343–52.

12 Holt IJ, Harding AE, Petty RK, *et al.* A new mitochondrial disease associated with mitochondrial DNA heteroplasmy. *Am J Hum Genet* 1990; **46**: 428–33.

This is partly based on a report originally published in *Neuromuscul Disord* 1995; **5(4)**: 345–6 with permission from Pergamon Press Ltd, Headington Hill Hall, Oxford OX3 0BW, UK.

19 Congenital Myasthenic Syndromes

LT Middleton *Cyprus Institute of Neurology and Genetics, Nicosia, Cyprus*

▶ Classification and Diagnostic Criteria

The term 'congenital myasthenic syndromes (CMS)' refers to a group of hereditary congenital disorders affecting the neuromuscular junction. These contrast with the auto-immune aetiology of myasthenia gravis and the Lambert–Eaton syndrome in which, respectively, antibodies to acetylcholine receptors (AChRs) and voltage-gated calcium channels are present in the majority of cases. Unlike the majority of other inherited neuromuscular diseases, little is, as yet, known of their molecular genetic mechanisms.

CMS have previously been classified according to the recognized site of the defect, i.e. presynaptic, postsynaptic or both[1]. In each of these groups, patients were further classified according to recognized effective mechanisms.

Two forms of **presynaptic CMS** have been identified, one due to a defect in ACH resynthesis of packaging[2], and the other two possibly of synaptic vesicles and/or reduced quantal release[3]. The former defect was found in one study with familial infantile myasthenia of autosomal recessive inheritance[4,5].

Congenital endplate acetylcholinesterase (AChE) **deficiency** was recognized in 1977 by Engel *et al.*[6] and four other cases were further reported[7].

Postynaptic defects involving the AChRs have been described with and without AChR deficiency on the basis of kinetic studies, as:

1 'Kinetic abnormalities of AChR with AChR deficiency' including the 'classic slow channel syndrome' as described by Engel *et al.*[8] and Oosterhuis *et al.*[9]; the 'Epsilon sub-unit mutations with prolonged open time and low conductance of the AChR channel'[10]; and 'AChR deficiency and short channel open time'[11].
2 'Kinetic abnormalities of AChR without AChR deficiency', observed in isolated cases by Engel. Two mechanisms were identified by Engel: 'high conductance fast-channel syndrome'[12] and a syndrome attributed to abnormal interaction of ACh with AChR[13].
3 Vincent *et al.*[14] and Bady *et al.*[15] showed that many patients examined in the UK had marked AChR deficiency associated with very abnormal endplate morphology, these changes being sufficient in themselves to account for the electrophysiological and clinical features of the disease. The inheritance in this form is probably autosomal recessive, though several cases have been sporadic.

Other forms of CMS have been reported in the literature. Vincent *et al.*[14] and Bady *et al.*[15] reported isolated patients with CMS resembling the Lambert–Eaton myasthenic syndrome and a small number of patients were found to have a 'familial limb girdle myasthenia'[16,17] of autosomal recessive inheritance. A benign form of CMS in oriental Jews with facial malformation was also reported[18].

Thus, clinical studies of CMS were limited to a very small number of laboratories in the world, where highly sophisticated morphological and electrophysiological techniques are available.

The following proposed classification and diagnostic criteria for congenital myasthenic syndromes are mainly based on clinical, genetic and neurophysiological features.

Classification

Type I autosomal recessive

Ia Familial infantile myasthenia.
Ib Limb girdle myasthenia.
Ic Acetylcholine esterase deficiency.
Id Acetylcholine receptor deficiency.

Type II autosomal dominant

IIa Slow channel syndrome.

Type III

Sporadic cases with no family history, excluding myasthenia gravis.

Congenital Myasthenic Syndromes Type Ia: Familial Infantile Myasthenia Syndrome

Clinical criteria

Mode of inheritance

Autosomal recessive.

Onset

From birth to early childhood, with fluctuating ptosis and involvement of bulbar muscles (poor cry and suck, feeding difficulties) and possible early respiratory distress.

Course

In childhood, symptoms and signs, of mild to moderate fatiguable weakness and variable ptosis and/or ophthalmoparesis. Occasional episodic exacerbations, usually precipitated by febrile illness and excitement, which may result in respiratory distress and apnoea. Subsequently, myasthenic symptoms and signs become less pronounced, with occurrence of mild to moderate fatiguable weakness of ocular, facial, bulbar or limb muscles.

Anticholinesterase medication

Usually improves symptoms and signs.

Associated symptoms and signs

Tendon reflexes remain normal. There is no atrophy, no signs of myopathy.

Laboratory criteria

1 Decremental response at 2–3 Hz stimulation in affected muscles, with the proviso that the decremental response may require studies to produce 'the exhaustion phenomenon' (prolonged exercise or repetitive stimulation at 3–5 Hz for 3 min).
2 Single fibre electromyography (SFEMG) abnormalities similar to those noted in myasthenia gravis, except that 'exhaustion' may be demonstrated during prolonged activation or axonal stimulation.

Exclusion criteria

1 Abnormal tendon reflexes or signs of atrophy/myopathy.
2 Progressive disease.
3 Presence of anti-AChR antibodies. Response to plasma exchange/immunosuppressive treatment.
4 Double CMAP responses to single nerve stimuli.

Congenital Myasthenic Syndromes Type Ib: Limb-Girdle Myasthenia Syndrome

Clinical criteria

Mode of inheritance

Autosomal recessive/sporadic

Onset

Usually in the teens.

Cardinal features

Symmetrical fatiguable weakness of limb-girdle muscles of the four limbs.

Laboratory criteria

1 Decremental response at 2–3 Hz repetitive stimulation.
2 Presence of tubular aggregates in muscle histochemistry.

Exclusion criteria

1 Involvement of ocular muscles.

2 Double CMAP evoked responses of single nerve stimuli.
3 Presence of anti-AChR antibodies. Response to plasma exchange/immunosuppressive treatment.

▶ Congenital Myasthenic Syndromes Type Ic: AChE Deficiency Syndrome

Clinical criteria

Mode of inheritance
Autosomal recessive.

Cardinal features
Onset at birth to the age of 2 years, with fatiguable weakness of facial, ocular and bulbar muscles. Delayed motor milestones
Selective involvement of axial muscles leading to fixed scoliosis in older patients
Slow pupillary responses to light
Symptoms refractory or worsened by anticholinesterase medication.

Additional features
Reduced tendon reflexes.

Laboratory criteria

1 Decremental response to repetitive nerve stimulation at 2–3 Hz, not corrected by Edrophonium.
2 Double CMAP evoked responses to single nerve stimuli.
3 Morphologic evidence of AChE deficiency using enzyme histochemical and/or immunocytochemical and/or double staining techniques.

Exclusion criteria

1 Improvement of symptoms by anticholinesterase medication.
2 Presence of anti-AChR antibodies. Response to plasma exchange/immunosuppressive treatment.

▶ Congenital Myasthenic Syndromes Type Id: AChR Deficiency Syndrome

Clinical criteria

Mode of inheritance
Autosomal recessive? but more common in males.

Onset
From birth or before 2 years with ptosis, bulbar muscle involvement and mild to moderate fatiguable weakness. No obvious exacerbating circumstances.

Course

Generally benign course but persists into adult life. Anti-AChE improves signs and symptoms. No atrophy or myopathy.

Laboratory criteria

Decremental response at 2–3 Hz, without exhaustion phenomenon. SFEMG abnormalities.

Optional inclusion criteria

AChE staining of endplates demonstrates abnormal elongation. AChR staining or binding studies demonstrates reduced AChR numbers.

Exclusion criteria

Presence of anti-AChR. Response to plasma exchange or immunosuppressive treatment. Double CMAP responses.

Congenital Myasthenic Syndromes Type IIa: Slow Channel Syndrome

Clinical criteria

Mode of inheritance

Autosomal dominant, with complete penetrance and variable expressivity. Rare sporadic cases.

Cardinal features

Variable age of onset, with fatiguable weakness of variable muscle distribution, and degree of severity. Progression is gradual or intermittent/stepwise with characteristic selective involvement of cranial and scapular muscles and the extensors of the hands and the fingers. Variable involvement of facial, ocular and bulbar muscles.

Additional features

Weakness and wasting of selectively affected muscles; reduced tendon reflexes.

Laboratory criteria

1 Double CMAP evoked responses to single nerve stimuli (constant).
2 Decremental response at 2–3 Hz repetitive nerve stimulation, in affected muscles.

Exclusion criteria

1 Absence of double CMAP response.
2 Presence of anti-AChR antibodies. Response to plasma exchange/immunosuppressive treatment.

Congenital Myasthenic Disorders Type III

To include all patients who demonstrate fatiguable weakness of a localized or generalized distribution, with age of onset before 12 years and neurophysiological evidence of neuromuscular transmission defect.

Exclusion criteria

1 Presence of anti-AChR or other specific antibodies.
2 Evidence of other CMS forms.
3 Response to plasma exchange or immunosuppression or other signs indicative of autoimmune aetiology.

References

1 Engel AG. Congenital myasthenic syndromes. In: Engel AG, Erduzini-Armstrong C, Eds. *Myology*. New York: McGraw-Hill, 1994; 1: 1806–35.
2 Mora M, Lambert EH, Engel AG. Synaptic vesicle abnormality in familial infantile myasthenia. *Neurology* 1987; **37**: 206–14.
3 Walls TJ, Engel AG, Nagel AS, *et al.* Congenital myasthenic syndrome associated with paucity of synaptic vesicles and reduced quantal release. *Ann NY Acad Sci* 1993; **681**: 461.
4 Robertson WC, Chun RWM, Kornguth SE. Familial infantile myasthenia. *Arch Neurol* 1980; **37**: 117–9.
5 Engel AG, Lambert EH. Congenital myasthenic syndromes. *Electroencephalogr Clin Neurophysiol Suppl* 1987; **39**: 91–102.
6 Engel AG, Lambert EH, Gomez MR. A new myasthenic syndrome with end-plate acetylcholinesterase deficiency, small nerve terminals, and reduced acetylcholine release. *Ann Neurol* 1977; **1**: 315–30.
7 Hutchinson DO, Walls TJ, Nakano S, *et al.* Congenital endplate acetylcholinesterase deficiency. *Brain* 1993; **116**: 633–53.
8 Engel AG, Lambert EH, Mulder DM, *et al.* A newly recognised congenital myasthenic syndrome attributed to a prolonged open time of the acetylcholine-induced ion channel. *Ann Neurol* 1982; **11**: 553–69.
9 Oosterhuis HJGH, Newsom-Davis J, Wokke JHJ, *et al.* The slow channel syndrome: two new cases. *Brain* 1987; **110**: 1061–78.
10 Engel AG, Hutchinson DO, Nakano S, *et al.* Myasthenic syndromes attributed to mutations affecting the epsilon subunit of the acetylcholine receptor. *Ann Acad Sci* 1993; **681**: 496–508.
11 Engel AG, Nagel A, Walls TJ, *et al.* Congenital myasthenic syndromes: I. Deficiency and short open-time of the acetylcholine receptor. *Muscle Nerve* 1993; **16**: 1284–92.

12 Engel AG, Uchitel O, Walls TJ, *et al.* Newly recognized congenital myasthenic syndrome associated with high conductance and fast closure of the acetylcholine receptor channel. *Ann Neurol* 1993; **34**: 38–47.

13 Uchitel O, Engel AG, Walls TJ, *et al.* Congenital myasthenic syndromes: II. A syndrome attributed to abnormal interaction of acetylcholine with its receptor. *Muscle Nerve* 1993; **16**: 1293–1301.

14 Vincent A, Newsom-Davis J, Wray D, *et al.* Clinical and experimental observations in patients with congenital myasthenic syndromes. *Ann NY Acad Sci* 1993; **681**: 451–60.

15 Bady B, Chauplannaz G, Carrier H. Congenital Lambert–Eaton myasthenic syndrome. *J Neurol Neurosurg Psychiatry* 1987; **50**: 476–8.

16 McQuillen MP. Familial limb-girdle myasthenia. *Brain* 1966; **89**: 121–32.

17 Vincent A, Cull-Candy S, Newsom-Davis J, *et al.* Congenital myasthenia: endplate acetylcholine receptors and electrophysiology in five cases. *Muscle Nerve* 1981; **4**: 306–18.

18 Bornstein B. Familial early myasthenia gravis. *Acta Paediatr* 1953; **42**: 442–7.

This is partly based on a report published in *Neuromuscul Disord* 1996; **6(2)**: 133–6 with permission from Pergamon Press Ltd, Headington Hill Hall, Oxford OX3 0BW, UK.

20 Post-polio Muscle Dysfunction

K Borg and J Borg *Dept of Neurology, Karolinska Hospital, Stockholm, Sweden*

E Stålberg *Dept of Clinical Neurophysiology, Uppsala University, Uppsala, Sweden*

▶ Diagnostic Criteria

Patients who have had poliomyelitis may experience more pronounced or new symptoms decades after the acute infection. These symptoms, also called late effects of polio, include unaccustomed fatigue, muscle and/or joint pain, new weakness in muscles previously affected or unaffected, new muscle atrophy, functional loss and cold intolerance. The condition has been named the **post-polio syndrome (PPS)** according to the clinical diagnostic criteria proposed by Halstead and Rossi[1]. The term **post-polio muscular atrophy** (PPMA) has been used for new muscle weakness and muscle atrophy[2], which were reported by more than 80% of a post-polio population[3]. In an isokinetic, five year follow-up study, 56% of the post-polio patients had developed increased or new muscle weakness at the second examination[4].

The 29th ENMC Workshop in 1994 was devoted to the neuromuscular symptoms of the late effects of poliomyelitis and an international consortium for research was founded[5]. There was a consensus among the participants that, based on neurophysiological and muscle biopsy data, most of the increased and new muscle weakness is due to ongoing denervation[5]. The denervation is compensated for by reinnervation and muscle fibre adaptation. Both these mechanisms are quite effective, but they have an upper limit. Further denervation, insufficient compensation and reduction of muscle fibre size lead to muscle weakness. The cause of the denervation is unknown[5].

In a large polio survey in Denmark, risk factors for developing late effects of polio were severity of paralysis and hospitalization during the acute infection. Current age and gender were confounding factors[6]. There is, on the basis of our knowledge today, no reason to believe that there is any genetic contribution to susceptibility to PPS.

The participants of the Workshop agreed that there was a need for diagnostic criteria primarily considering the neuromuscular symptoms of PPS. The term **post-polio muscle dysfunction (PPMD)** was proposed with the following clinical and laboratory criteria:

Clinical criteria

I History of paralytic polio.
I After a period of functional stability for at least 15 years development of new muscle dysfunction. Muscle weakness and/or muscle atrophy and/or muscle pain and/or muscle fatigue.
I Neurological examination compatible with prior poliomyelitis.
Muscle weakness, muscle atrophy, and decreased or absent tendon reflexes compatible with a lower motor neuron lesion.
No sensory loss.
C Signs of generalized neuropathy **exclude** the diagnosis. Sensory loss limited to a certain dermatome or to a peripheral nerve territory due to compression of nerve roots or peripheral nerves **does not exclude** the diagnosis.

Laboratory criteria

I Neurophysiological examination with findings compatible with prior poliomyelitis. Signs of reinnervation on electromyography but no signs of polyneuropathy.
I Muscle biopsy and/or magnetic resonance imaging (MRI) with findings compatible with prior poliomyelitis. Neuropathic histopathological abnormalities in muscle biopsy are compatible with prior poliomyelitis but are also found in other neurogenic conditions. Secondary myopathic abnormalities may be seen in advanced cases of prior poliomyelitis. Both muscle biopsy and MRI may add diagnostic information for inclusion and also for exclusion, but the examinations are not required for the diagnosis.

References

1 Halstead LS, Rossi CD. Post-polio syndrome: Clinical experience with 132 consecutive outpatients. In: *Research and clinical aspects of the late effects of poliomyelitis*. Halstead LS, Wiechers DO, Eds. Birth defects: Original Article Series 1987; **23(4)**: 13–26.
2 Dalakas MC, Sever JL, Madden DL, *et al.* Late post-poliomyelitis muscular atrophy: Clinical virologic and immunologic study. *Rev Infect Dis* 1984; **6 (Suppl 2)**: S562–7.
3 Ahlström G, Gunnarsson LG, Leissner P, *et al.* Epidemiology of neuromuscular diseases. Including the post-polio sequelae, in a Swedish county. *Neuroepidemiol* 1993; **12**: 262–9.
4 Grimby G, Hedberg M, Henning GB. Changes in muscle morphology, strength and enzymes in a 4–5 year follow-up of subjects with poliomyelitis sequelae. *Scand J Rehab Med* 1994; **26**: 121–30.
5 Borg K. Workshop report. Post-polio muscle dysfunction. 29th ENMC Workship 14–16 October 1994, Naarden, The Netherlands. *Neuromuscul Disord* 1996; **6**: 75–80.
6 Lønnberg F. Late onset polio sequelae in Denmark. Presentation and results of a nation-wide survey of 3607 polio survivors. *Scand J Rehab Med* 1993; **28 (Supp 28)**: 7–15.

This is based on a report originally published in *Neuromuscul Disord* 1996; **6(1)**: 75–80 with permission from Pergamon Pres Ltd, Headington Hill Hall, Oxford OX3 OBW, UK.

Index

Note: As this book is set out with disease/disorder headings followed by diagnostic criteria and laboratory investigations, the index is confined to main headings and variants with only occasional further detail where considered necessary.